HOW NOT TO
DROP DEAD!

HOW NOT TO DROP DEAD!

A GUIDE FOR PREVENTION OF 201 CAUSES OF SUDDEN OR RAPID DEATH

Eduardo Chapunoff, M.D., F.A.C.P., F.A.C.C.

Library of Congress Control Number: 2009901551
ISBN: Hardcover   978-1-4415-1357-1
               Softcover   978-1-4415-1356-4

www.dreduardochapunoff.com
E-mail: eduardochapunoff@bellsouth.net

Library of Congress Cataloging-in-Publication Data

How Not to Drop Dead! A Guide for Prevention of 201 Causes of Sudden or Rapid Death/Eduardo Chapunoff

Includes Index

Illustrations by Dr. Eduardo Chapunoff

The author and the publisher assume no responsibility for errors, inaccuracies, omissions, or any other inconsistency herein. Likewise, they assume no responsibility for any consequences any person might suffer from following concepts described in this book. This publication is only an educational guide and does not provide medical treatments. Readers are urged to consult their physicians and follow their advice.

This book was printed in the United States of America.

To order additional copies of this book, contact:
Xlibris Corporation
1-888-795-4274
www.Xlibris.com
Orders@Xlibris.com
32887

CONTENTS

DEDICATION

This book is dedicated to firefighters
and fire-rescue workers who often risk their own lives
to avoid the sudden or rapid death of others.

ACKNOWLEDGMENTS

I want to express my deepest gratitude to my wife Maria Cristina for the poetry, love, and joy she instilled into my life.

I extend my profound appreciation to the senior executives of the Doctor's Medical Center, Miami, Dr. Ventura de Paz, President and CEO, Luis Portal, Vice-President, Dr. Anel Monrose, General Manager, Kenia Cancio, Assistant Manager, and Magaly Castaneda, Director, Human Resources, for the immense support they've given me to perform my professional duties. I admire their effectiveness, integrity, and sensitivity. I can't find the right words to describe the affection and respect I have for them.

I also wish to convey my recognition to Dr. Patrick Gray, Medical Director and Dr. Augusto Cruz Garcia for their special collaboration and all of the administrative and health-care employees at the Doctor's Medical Center, for making my life easier and happier every day.

My eternal thanks go to the memory of my parents Julio and Jacinta. If anything good ever came out of me, it's all due to them.

Eduardo Chapunoff

EXCERPTS FROM REVIEWS AND QUOTES ON

ANSWERING YOUR QUESTIONS ABOUT HEART DISEASE AND SEX

Eduardo Chapunoff, M.D.

Foreword by

Arnold A. Lazarus, Ph.D.
Distinguished Professor Emeritus of Psychology
Rutgers University

EDITOR'S CHOICE
iUniverse

FINALIST
ForeWord Magazine's 2004 Book of the Year Awards

"Mental Health professionals and professionals in training . . . Here is a book that gives information, compassion, and how-to in an easy read for you and your patients. A sensitive topic ever so elegantly handled."

-Judith Coche, Ph.D.
Director, the Coche Center, New Jersey and Pennsylvania

**

"A book written with humoristic and didactic brilliance."

-Frank Perez-Rivas
Ret. Director, Oakland Park Veterans Administration Clinic, Oakland Park, Florida

**

"This book takes the mystique out of heart disease. Chapunoff doesn't hold back on the humor—not a bad idea, considering the gravity under which some readers might be studying this book."

"With fifty-nine million Americans suffering from cardiovascular diseases, this text has the potential for becoming a well-thumbed reference book."

-Karl Kunkel
Critic, ForeWord Magazine

**

"The author provides a knowledgeable and caring approach to an important new topic. Highly recommended!"

-Raymond C. Rosen, Ph.D.
Professor of Psychiatry and Medicine, Robert Wood Johnson Medical School, New Jersey
Director of Human Sexuality Program

**

"Any literate individual with an interest in his or her health, and specifically anyone who wants to know more about love, life, hearts, sex, compassion, and human relationships, will find this book of enormous value. Professionals can also derive benefit from Dr. Chapunoff's vast experience and profound wisdom."

"This book makes me feel with all my heart that Dr. Chapunoff was my personal physician."

Arnold A. Lazarus, Ph.D.
Distinguished Professor Emeritus of Psychology, Rutgers University, New Jersey

**

"Dr. Chapunoff succeeds with the professional maturity that comes from years of experience listening to his patients from all walks of life. A provocative sense of humor makes the reading fun."

"I have not seen a more inspiring and integrative work on the connections between health, intimacy, and happiness. This book is a true celebration of the human heart and spirit."

-Dr. Scott E. Borrelli, Ed.D., Clinical Psycho.
Collegiate Professor, The University of Maryland European Division
Director of Counseling Services. The American Intercontinental University of London

**

"Dr. Chapunoff uses an intriguing, comfortable, and witty format to address intimate health issues. There are no other books addressing the issues he covers. He is honest and fortright with his answers."

"This excellent resource proves that an informative and educational reading experience can also be engaging, even when the subject matter is very serious."

-Betty Corbin Tucker
Nationwide television and radio appearances. Past Editor of a nationally distributed magazine. Conductor of writing seminars.

**

"Dr. Chapunoff's superb book is a godsend for the 59 million Americans who have cardiovascular disease. With its easy to understand writing style, its poignant clinical vignettes, its solid medical advice, and a superb index, this book deserves to be widely read and recommended."

Aline Zoldbrod, Ph.D.
Sex Therapist, Boston, Massachusetts
Author of *Sex Smart*—ForeWord Magazine award winner
Co-Author of *Sex Talk*

**

"This book is of value to anyone who has a sex drive and a beating heart!"

-Jackqueline Sousa
Editor—Coral Gables Living
President, Metropical Media Corp., Coral Gables, Florida

**

"This book is a fun, interesting read employing a lot of humor and great anecdotes. And it's got to be a more fun and relevant read for a cardiac patient than the week-old Better Homes & Gardens in the hospital room. Forget the twenty-dollar get-well bouquet: give your convalescent a sex life for $ 15,95."

-John Huetter
Critic, Boca Raton News, Boca Raton, Florida

**

"Dr. Chapunoff offers the balm of simple clarity, compassion, and rock-solid guidance. There's a reason Dr. Chapunoff is held in such high regard . . . his skill, his writing, and his guidance are totally approachable, gentle, and wise!"

"Bravo to Doctors such as Eduardo, a true, loving healer!"

-Bernie Ahearn
Radio Host of A Man's World, Detroit, Michigan

**

"I liked this book. It was informative without being preachy, straightforward and not so technical that it went over my head. By discussing things in a straghtforward manner, readers will find there is little to be embarrassed about. Humor is generously sprinkled to assist in the process".

-Nancy Gail
BC Books, Georgia

**

"Upbeat, direct, straightforward conversational style. Dr. Chapunoff is a master of knowing how to pull in his readers by presenting information that is current and relevant".

Norm Goldman
Editor and Publisher of Books for Pleasure, Montreal, Canada

FIGURES

INTRODUCTION

Death is the only examination we all pass without ever studying for it.

Death is a common phenomenon. I'm sure you've noticed. Evidently, it is also a worrisome phenomenon, judging by what most people think of it.

We can't avoid death, but if we are careful and lucky, we can hope for a postponement, a sort of negotiated settlement with destiny.

A logical death, whatever that is, makes sense, and I'd vote for it. Perhaps we should consider a logical death—the kind of demise where relatives and friends grieve the loss but do not consider it to be utterly senseless: a long battle with cancer, a severe stroke with total disability including blindness and deafness, and having advanced dementia at old age.

Many deaths, though, are illogical. They don't make sense and shouldn't happen. From my own perspective, a death that doesn't make sense is a death that could have been prevented.

In the course of this book, you'll become aware of many different causes of sudden or rapid death. And when you see how easily some of them could have been avoided, you'll be tempted to pull your hair and verbalize your disappointment and frustration.

One finds it more acceptable to deal with loss of life that involved a struggle for survival, a fight against a disease. But meeting death at the corner of the next block because of negligence, carelessness, ignorance, or sloppiness is particularly sad. And at times, if you allow me to be totally candid and frank about it, it's also kind of stupid.

DEATH AND CIVILIZATIONS

History has recorded innumerable instances of people who died gladly—and painfully—with a radical conviction, at the stake; by hanging; at the Roman circus; the guillotine; or had their bodies mutilated or perforated through and through by a bullet, an arrow, or the spade in duels and battlefields, for love, honor, riches, power ambitions, or loyalty to a revolutionary sociopolitical idea, a religious faith, a commander or a king, who, incidentally, more often than not, took that kind of sacrifice as expected and granted and made nothing out of it.

The glamour claimed with certain heroic deaths doesn't necessarily make the process of dying more appealing or attractive to most people.

Generally speaking, death is not a particularly welcome event. People die because they have to, not because they like it. But there are always exceptions for everything, death included, of course: take the case of the suicide bombers. They have no fear and are elated about their decision.

But then, there are those who commit suicide because of severe depression and are unable to find a way out of their misery. That is unfortunate for a number of reasons; one of them being the fact that many self-induced fatalities could be avoided by timely diagnosis and effective treatment of a gloomy state of mind. You'd be surprised to know how many individuals who have suicidal intentions and have made an attempt to kill themselves changed their minds and had a zest for life after receiving appropriate therapy.

In the Western culture, there's a sense of rebellion about death. Even elderly people are anxious to live a little—or a lot—longer.

Deeply religious individuals handle their spiritual affairs differently—and more effectively. They are assertive, confident, and they accept death with resignation and even contentment, thinking that they'll soon be in a painless world, together with their God, their beloved parents, children, wives, mistresses, lovers, relatives, friends, and pets, depending upon their individual taste and preferences.

Religious conviction certainly makes a difference: those who expect the Lord to give them mercy and a place in heaven are very fortunate. Not only they believe they'll live in the afterlife, but that they'll live happily forever. Can't beat that!

For those who suffer extraordinary physical or psychological pains, death may represent a solution, not a problem. It puts an end to their agony and torment.

I've witnessed the process of dying many times. Commonly, people die unaware of their passing and are often unresponsive, obtunded, or comatose. Others remain alert up to the last moment.

WITNESSING THE ACT OF DYING

Years ago I was treating and watching a dying man, who was struggling to catch his breath. His lungs were filled with fluid. He was ninety, fully alert to the end and had been a very dear patient of mine for twenty years. Bill knew the end was near. He was a sweet man. And a wise man too. We used to chat about life during his visits to my office. He'd say, "Ed, don't worry! If you want to enjoy life, live for a long time, and be at peace with yourself, remember this: *Never worry!*"

Moments before he died he saw me struggling to control my tears and grabbed my hand with his. It was amazingly strong for an agonizing person. He looked straight at my eyes, and said to me what he had always said, "Ed, remember: Never worry!" Then he closed his eyes and passed away.

Bill was going through such a difficult situation, and yet, he was the one who offered the consolation. At age ninety and fully aware of his imminent passing, he had more courage than I did. What a beautiful and inspiring man he was!

This is the kind of experience you never forget. I just hope that when my time is up, I'll be able to display, at least, half of his charm, courage, and wisdom.

The process of dying can be acute, chronic, or anything in between. Many people die slowly. Others do it fast. A proportion of them die even faster: they died suddenly. Those who expire quickly will be the subject of this book.

Sudden death can be painless if it occurs during natural sleep or induced by general anesthesia. It's the kind of death that most humans would love to subscribe to.

Rapid demises may at times be a nightmare. One example is the choking that results from having a piece of food lodging in the respiratory tract instead of having gone through the natural esophageal (food pipe) route. There's a way to treat this condition, and I've described it in this book (please see Heimlich maneuver).

DEFINITION OF SUDDEN DEATH

Cardiologists define *sudden death* as the termination of life in one hour's time. Coroners and pathologists extend the concept of sudden death to a demise that takes place in less than twenty-four hours. I'll be discussing examples of both. Some of the deaths I listed and discussed in the book occur in a few days. After all, the loss of a life in such a short period of time should not be categorized as a "slow death." So I consider the decision to incorporate them here, justified.

DIFFERENT KINDS OF SUDDEN DEATH

- **Natural:** death is the result of a disease
- **Suicidal:** death caused by self, with conscious intent
- **Homicidal:** death caused by another human
- **Accidental:** unintended death, not resulting from a natural, suicidal, or homicidal cause
- **Undetermined:** no evidence to justify the cause of death is found

WAYS OF AVOIDING SUDDEN DEATH

- **Prevention:** taking precautions to avoid illnesses and accidents
- **Treatment:** dealing with an emergency at the time of its occurrence

Some sudden deaths can be prevented. Others cannot. Take the case of an airplane that crashes in a populated area on top restaurants, banks, and people walking in the street. Who in this world could prevent such a disaster?

Other forms of sudden death can be avoided. Many preventable actions can be deployed against smoking, obesity, hypertension, high blood levels of cholesterol and triglycerides, sedentary lifestyles, and stress among others. The consequences of neglecting these cardiovascular risk factors may be a sudden death, but the methodical deployment of defective lifestyles that will eventually cause a sudden departure from this world may take decades.

Many heart attacks, strokes, heart failure, ruptured aneurysms or massive pulmonary embolus (a large clot blocking the pulmonary artery and originating in a leg vein), and many other disorders that culminate in sudden or rapid death could be avoided by the application of healthy habits, also defined as **prevention**, the ideal solution, **or by their early detection and treatment**, the second best alternative.

Early detection and treatment of a disease is often lifesaving, but **given the choice, choose prevention.**

Other sudden deaths result from the use of illicit substances such as cocaine, heroin, and other popular drugs in all-night dance parties, such as ecstasy. In a few minutes, the victims—often teenagers or young adults—become part of gloomy statistics.

Aging is a risk factor but affects every person in a different way. Illnesses associated with advanced age make a big difference. So it isn't only age that matters, but what comes along with it.

Genes cannot be changed although at times they make room for negotiation: an example is the cerebral aneurysm, a focal dilatation of a cerebral artery that always carries the risk of rupture. There are members of a family who carry cerebral aneurysms. So the presence of a cerebral aneurysm may be inevitable, but its detection and treatment allows its correction before it bursts. Once it does, it's very difficult to avoid a fatal outcome.

The number of causes of sudden or rapid death is so impressive that I couldn't have mentioned them in this book. Keep in mind that this book is not an Encyclopedia but a Guide. I've briefly described 201, hoping that by reminding you of their existence and ways to prevent them, one day you could save your life or the life of another person.

There's something sacred about life. Any person who contributes to save another human being or prevent a tragedy, regardless of his/her profession, derives a kind of spiritual satisfaction that cannot be compared with anything else.

You may think you need to be a trained professional of the health care field to prevent a sudden death. Sometimes you do. Sometimes you don't! Obviously, the better trained a person is in medical emergencies, the greater the chances that a victim's life will be saved.

Ironically, a cardiac arrest may be resolved by an inexperienced witness with little knowledge of cardiopulmonary resuscitation: 911 arrives at the scene in a couple of minutes, the victim is taken to the hospital and survives without complications. Other times, a person has a cardiac arrest in front of experienced professionals in resuscitation techniques, and their combined efforts fail to revive the victim.

HOW TO APPROACH THE READING OF THIS BOOK

This work contains a lot of information. It isn't the type of book you can read and assimilate overnight. It's probably better to start by focusing on the subjects that apply to your particular situation or interest.

If you or a person you care about suffers from heart disease, you may want to read that section as well as cardiovascular risk factors first. If you have asthma and you're allergic to drugs, bee stings, or environmental allergies, I recommend you to read first the chapters on anaphylaxis (acute life-threatening allergic reaction), bee stings, and asthma. If you like to swim in the ocean, read the section on shark attacks and the one on drowning. If you have a first degree relative who had a cerebral aneurysm or you learned about someone who died of sepsis, carbon monoxide poisoning, suicide, anorexia, asphyxia, sudden infant death, heart failure during pregnancy, acute alcoholic intoxication, cocaine use or abuse, electrocution, morbid obesity, or died during sexual activity or doing scuba diving, review these areas of personal interest before you approach others.

While reading this work, always think that anything that can produce a rapid or sudden death listed here has the potential to affect you or someone you love. If those who lost their lives in a manner that could have been prevented had the capacity to tell us about their experience,

I'm sure that some of them would tell us: *"You know what? I never thought that this could happen to me!"*

Many rapid or sudden deaths are tragedies, but more so when they could have been prevented. This book flashes a light of warning. I mentioned 201 causes of rapid or sudden demise, but there are many more that were omitted. In the Epilogue, I explain why.

And now that you're about to become more familiar with the broad spectrum of potentially catastrophic sudden and rapid demises, if the exposure and analysis of so many deadly events makes you sad and excessively preoccupied, at least every fifteen minutes, think more about life and living than about death and dying.

PART 1

ANEURYSMS

The ruthless executioners.

In the course of my career, I saw a number of aneurysms in different locations of the human body. Those that ruptured, regardless of the arterial territory involved, were all unforgettable experiences. The presentations were always acute, intense, dramatic. Do you remember the TV series or movies dealing with medical emergencies at a hospital where medical personnel run in all directions trying to get things done at the maximum speed? Well, ruptured aneurysms meant all that . . . and more.

An aneurysm is a focal dilatation of an artery. The word *aneurysm* comes from the Greek *aneurysma*, meaning "widening." Aneurysms develop in multiple territories. When an aneurysm bursts in the brain or the aorta, life is in extremely serious danger.

There is one kind of aneurysm that is not a focal dilatation of an artery but a portion of the left ventricle that suffered a myocardial infarction. The heart muscle is replaced by scar tissue that has no contractile power. This "useless" area bulges out every time the heart contracts, and it is called left ventricular aneurysm, and we'll describe it later on in this section.

The normal aorta arises at the level of the aortic valve and is divided into three segments: ascending aorta, aortic arch, and descending aorta.

AORTIC ANEURYSMS

These usually occur because the wall of the artery has been damaged and weakened by atherosclerotic plaques. Sometimes, there are no such plaques, and the aneurysm results from a weakness of the mid-layer of the aortic wall, which may or may not be congenital. When it is of congenital origin, it is called the Marfan syndrome.

The pressure inside the arterial system pushes the aortic wall outward, and this results in the formation of an aneurysm. Hypertension facilitates the process. The aneurysm's size may remain stationary for years or grow to the breaking point.

Besides **"rupture,"** there's another way for the aneurysm to create an acute crisis: that is **"dissection."** Here the blood leaks along the wall of the artery. Incidentally, dissection may occur in the presence or absence of an aneurysm.

Commonest risk factors that trigger the formation of an aneurysm:

Acquired	**Congenital**
* Atherosclerosis	* Marfan syndrome
* Hypertension	
* Smoking	

Other contributing risk factors: age older than fifty-five, male, family history (a first degree relative also had aneurysm), Caucasian, high cholesterol levels, trauma (falls and motor vehicle accidents, and syphilis.

1—ABDOMINAL AORTIC ANEURYSM (AAA)

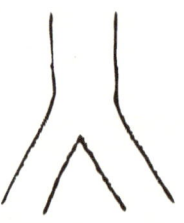   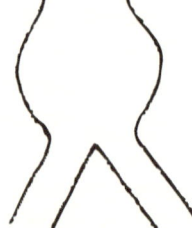

A—Normal abdominal aorta   B—Abdominal aortic aneurysm (AAA)

Figure 1

The characteristic symptoms are low back and abdominal pain. **Sometimes, an AAA expands and gives no symptoms.**

Palpation of your abdomen by the doctor may or may not disclose an AAA. If you have a thin, easily palpable abdomen, the examining physician can feel it. If your belly is obese, the professional cannot detect it. A quick and simple test, the abdominal aortic ultrasound, will often show it.

TREATMENT

If the aneurysm is small, you will be recommended a periodic evaluation of its size. At this stage, that's generally done once a year.

An aneurysm that causes symptoms must be treated. Surgery is recommended for aneurysms bigger than 5.5 cm in width. Many doctors take that approach when the AAA reached 5 cm in diameter, or when the size is smaller, but it has quickly increased its size (see a few lines below).

Unruptured AAA Treatment Approach

The traditional open repair. A large cut is made in the abdomen, and the aneurysm is replaced with a graft made of synthetic material, such as Dacron.

The endovascular stent. Not all unruptured AAA can be treated by this method. This is indicated for AAA located below the renal arteries or aortic aneurysms having the following:

* Adequate access to the arteries of the groin (iliac-femoral arteries)
* AAA diameter less than 5 cm
* AAA diameter of 4-5 cm, which has also increased in size by 0.5 cm in the last six months or 1 cm for the last twelve months
* Aneurysm which is twice the diameter of the normal infrarenal aorta

Ruptured AAA

This needs emergent surgical repair. Blood rushes into the abdominal cavity, and the patient quickly goes into shock.

A retired physician in his seventies felt that something inside his abdomen "was going to burst." He was markedly obese. An immediate evaluation revealed a large AAA (12 cm in width). During surgery, the AAA was seen rubbing against the spine; its wall was getting eroded, and it was ready to burst. He had a full recovery.

—*—

Years ago, and in a two-week period, I was called to see two elderly men (both in the eighties), who arrived at the emergency department in shock, severely anemic, and with a large testicle simulating a hernia. It wasn't a hernia. One testicular area was filled up with blood that had come from a ruptured AAA and had descended into the testicle. The anemia was due to the massive intra-abdominal bleeding. One of these patients was attempted a surgical repair but expired post-operatively due to severe heart failure. The second one died minutes after his arrival to the emergency room.

2—AORTIC DISSECTION

This is an infrequent but often fatal condition. In September 2007 it killed the award-winning actor John Ritter. It also killed King George II of England; Richard Biggs, actor; Mike Wieringo, American comic book artist; Jonathan Larson, composer of *Rent*; and the unforgettable Lucille Ball. Who can forget her and the *I Love Lucy* show?

But some were fortunate enough to survive aortic dissection. The eminent cardiovascular surgeon, Dr. Michael DeBakey, who created surgical methods to treat aortic dissection in addition to a host of other cardiovascular techniques, ran into trouble when he developed his own aortic dissection at age ninety-seven in February 2006. He not only survived the operation, but he went back to work. Dr. DeBakey died in 2008 at the age of ninety-nine.

I recently saw a forty-eight-year-old black female who had a history of long-standing hypertension with a dissecting descending aorta aneurysm. She presented with severe upper abdominal pain radiated to the left scapular area. She was treated medically and survived the ordeal. A month later, she complained of a few episodes of mild left scapular discomfort. A CT angiogram showed a recurrence and worsening of the descending aorta dissection, and she was urgently and successfully treated with a stent.

Approximately 10,000 Americans suffer from aortic dissections each year. **This is a tear in the wall of the aorta due to its midlayer collagen degeneration that forces the blood to flow between the layers of the wall of the aorta and leads to the layers separation.** This disease often presents with intolerable chest pain and carries a mortality of 80%. Fifty percent of patients die before reaching the hospital.

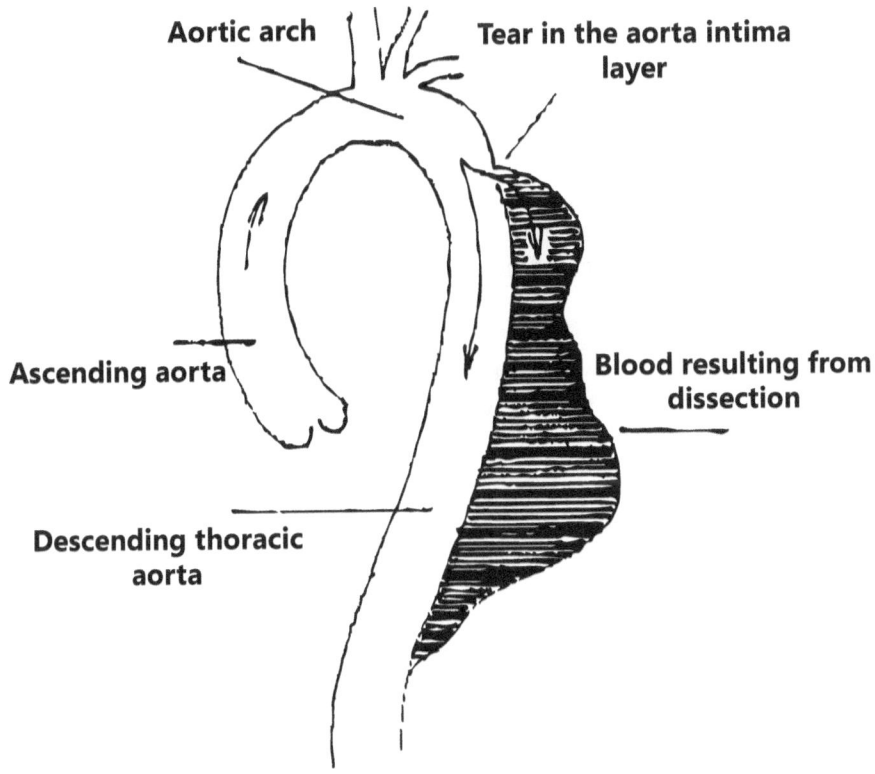

Aortic dissection

Figure 2

The highest incidence of aortic dissection occurs in persons aged 50-70. This condition is associated with hypertension, connective tissue disorders, or a blunt injury to the thorax, usually a car accident, but may also occur following aortic valve replacement or in those who were inserted an intra-aortic balloon pump for the treatment of shock.

Half of the dissections in women before forty occur during pregnancy and usually in the third trimester.

The diagnosis is established by computed tomography, CT, MRI, trans-esophageal echocardiography, and aortogram. The latter involves placement of a catheter in the aorta and injection of contrast material while taking x-rays.

The risk of death is highest in the first few hours after the dissection begins. Some of the aortic dissections are not that lethal. If the patient survives for a couple of weeks, there's a better outlook.

Treatment approach depends upon the location of the dissection. If this involves the ascending aorta, surgical management is superior to medical management. When more distal portions of the aorta are affected, including the abdominal aorta, medical management is the preferred approach.

One critical aspect of the treatment of a dissecting aortic aneurysm is the use of medications to control hypertension: aortic dissection gets worse when the blood pressure is elevated.

3—AORTIC ANEURYSM, ASCENDING AORTA AND AORTIC ARCH ANEURYSM

Symptoms depend on the type and location of the aneurysm and result from pressure caused by aneurysm pressing against organs, nerves, and other blood vessels.

shortness of breath
hoarseness
dry cough
pulsating pain in the chest or head

4—AORTIC ANEURYSM, DESCENDING THORACIC AORTA

Symptoms: Pain in the left shoulder, chest wall, or in between shoulder blades.

TREATMENT OF ASCENDING, AORTIC ARCH, AND DESCENDING AORTA ANEURYSMS

It depends on the location of the aneurysm.

Aneurysm of the Ascending Aorta or Aortic Arch

Surgery to replace the aorta is recommended if the aneurysm is larger than 5-6 cm. This is done with a Dacron graft (a fabric substitute).

Aneurysm of the Descending Thoracic Aorta

Option 1: If it is larger than 6 cm, major **surgery** is required to replace the aorta.

Option 2: Endovascular stenting is a less-invasive alternative. A stent is a tiny metal or plastic tube that is passed through a catheter inserted in the groin and is placed into the aneurysm.

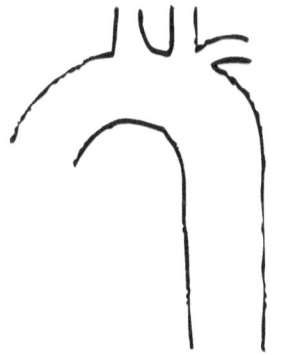 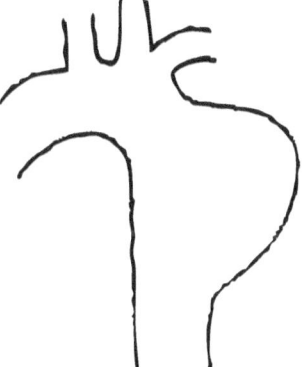

A—Normal thoracic aorta   B—Aneurysm, descending thoracic aorta

Figure 3

5—CEREBRAL ARTERY ANEURYSM ("BERRY" ANEURYSM)

A **cerebral, intracranial, or "berry" aneurysm** is an abnormal bulge, like a bubble, in a brain artery. It develops in a small, weakened area of a blood vessel.

A small, stable aneurysm will produce no symptoms. When its size increases, it may remain symptom free or produce symptoms before it ruptures: severe headaches, nausea and vomiting, vision impairment, and loss of consciousness.

Unfortunately, brain aneurysms are often discovered at the worst possible time, and that is, when they burst. This means bleeding into the brain, brain damage, and death. The majority of cerebral aneurysms rupture without preceding symptoms.

About 4% of young adults and up to 10% of elderly patients have cerebral aneurysms. Rupture occurs in 65-75% of patients, usually before age fifty.

Over 30,000 people in the United States annually develop this complication. Following the aneurysm rupture, 12% of those affected die before reaching the hospital, and over 50% will die within the first thirty days.

Size of the Aneurysms

Cerebral aneurysms vary in size from less than 15 mm (small) to 15 to 25 mm (large), 25 to 50 mm (giant), and over 50 mm (supergiant).

Causes of Development of Brain Aneurysms: congenital tendency, smoking, blood infections localizing germs in a cerebral artery, brain injury, hypertension.

Diagnosis of Unruptured Aneurysm

It's done by magnetic resonance imaging (MRI), magnetic resonance angiography (MRA), and computed tomography angiography (CTA). A cerebral angiogram provides more definitive information.

Screening for cerebral aneurysms using the tests just mentioned **is recommended for those who are at a high risk of having them,** such as those with a **significant family history of brain aneurysms and those who suffer from polycystic kidney disease (multiple cysts of different sizes in both kidneys).**

Diagnosis of a Ruptured Aneurysm

The main tests to diagnose this condition are the following:

- *Computarized tomography (CT).* This is an x-ray technique that examines the brain in cross-sectional slices
- *Cerebrospinal fluid examination.* A needle is inserted into the lower back to obtain a small amount of cerebrospinal fluid. If this contains blood, it means blood reached the subarachnoid space (this is the space that exists between the brain and its surrounding membrane called "the subarachnoid membrane")
- *Cerebral angiography.* All patients with a diagnosis of subarachnoid hemorrhage or in whom an aneurysm is suspected require **cerebral angiography.** This test is essential since it provides critical information about size, shape, and location of the aneurysm in addition to the diagnosis of vasospasm, a constriction of a brain artery that should be treated aggressively to prevent additional brain damage

Treatment of unruptured cerebral aneurysm: the goal of treatment is prevention of future cerebral hemorrhage.

Treatment of ruptured cerebral aneurysm: the goal of treatment is to stop the brain hemorrhage.

Both of the above are done in two ways:

- Neurosurgery
- Endovascular surgery

Neurosurgery: Clipping of the aneurysm. It involves general anesthesia. An incision in the scalp creates a window. The aneurysm is located, and its neck is obliterated with a metallic clip. The operation then requires direct exposure of the brain and the aneurysm.

Endovascular surgery. Endovascular coiling consists of passing a catheter into the femoral artery in the groin, is advanced through the aorta, and reaches the brain arteries and finally the aneurysm itself. Platinum coils are pushed into the aneurysm and released. These initiate a clotting reaction within the aneurysm that, if successful, will eliminate the aneurysm.

To sum it up: Prevent the rupture of a cerebral aneurysm by detecting it before it causes symptoms or when there are early signs indicating its possible presence, such as headaches or other neurological deficits.

6—CORONARY ARTERY ANEURYSM

This abnormality is always found in an angiogram when the cardiologist is looking for something else. And then surfaces the inevitable question: should it be treated, or should it be left alone?

This is an uncommon disease. It is defined as a focal coronary artery dilatation that exceeds the diameter of the patient's largest coronary vessel by 1.5-2 times. Sometimes, coronary artery aneurysms can be large. A coronary artery aneurysm measuring 6 x 8 cm has been reported.

The natural course of a coronary artery aneurysm, its outlook or prognosis, and even what to do about it once it is diagnosed remain uncertain. Atherosclerosis is responsible for the majority of coronary aneurysms.

This kind of aneurysm can produce symptoms of angina or acute myocardial infarction by forming a clot inside the aneurysm (thrombus) or releasing that clot into the coronary artery.

Management varies. Some cardiac surgeons favor its resection and using a vein of the leg to join the healthy segments of the left coronary artery. Others prefer not to touch it.

7—LEFT VENTRICULAR ANEURYSM

This is a piece of dead heart muscle that develops as follows:

If the blockage of a coronary artery leads to an acute myocardial infarction, the damaged or dead heart muscle is no longer cardiac muscle but scar tissue. This area does not contract per se. It moves because it is pulled by the surrounding heart muscle, and it bulges out every time the heart contracts. This bulging area is a left ventricular aneurysm. Its presence diminishes the capacity of the heart to eject normal amount of blood into the general circulation, and this may translate into **heart failure**

The left ventricular aneurysm may also generate **life-threatening arrhythmias,** and **clots** are occasionally formed inside the bulging sac. These are sometimes released into the arterial system.

A left ventricular aneurysm can be surgically removed, and this is usually combined with coronary bypass with very good results.

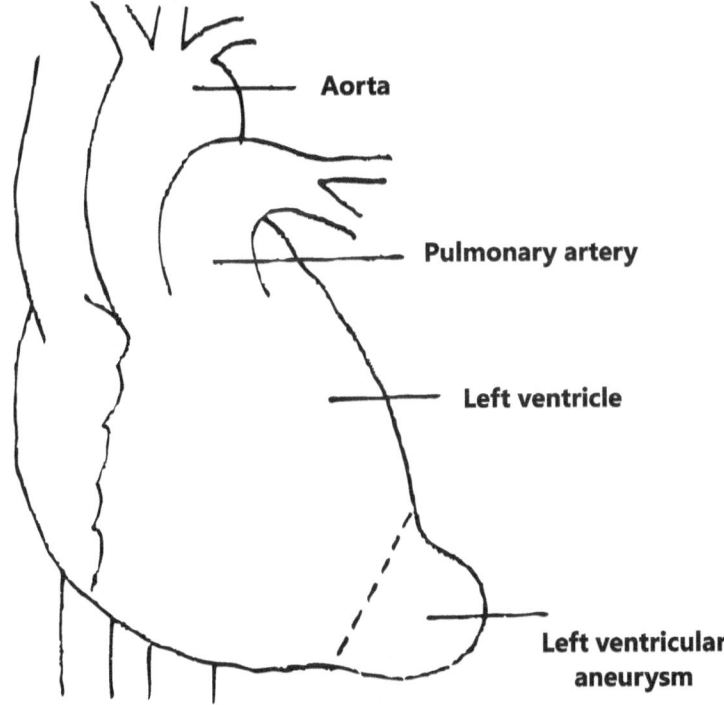

Aorta

Pulmonary artery

Left ventricle

Left ventricular aneurysm

Left ventricular aneurysm following a myocardial infarction

Figure 4

8—LEFT VENTRICULAR PSEUDOANEURYSM

In a true left ventricular aneurysm, part of the left ventricular muscle is replaced by scar tissue, but the wall of the left ventricle has not ruptured. A left ventricular pseudoaneurysm occurs when there is a myocardial infarction, and a little opening in the heart muscle develops (small perforation), and blood enters the pericardial space. It can be diagnosed by echocardiography, nuclear study of the left ventricle, and/or MRI.

Surgery is a must in all cases of left ventricular pseudoaneurysm.

A sixty-five-year-old businessman living in Venezuela appeared in terminal condition due to heart failure. His wife and brother, who was a physician, made arrangements for his funeral. In a desperate move he was brought to Miami Beach and became my patient. He looked critically ill, could barely catch his breath, and his whole body was massively edematous: his lower extremities and abdomen showed huge amounts of fluid retention. We thought he wouldn't probably survive an emergent cardiac catheterization, but he did. He was immediately taken to surgery. He had sustained a myocardial infarction that contained a small area of rupture or perforation of the left ventricular wall that had leaked blood into the pericardium. Luckily, a corklike blood clot had blocked the little hole and that avoided a massive passage of blood from the left ventricular cavity into the pericardium. He was repaired the left ventricle opening and drained the pericardial blood and fully recovered. He went back to Venezuela, and three months after his treatment in Florida, he was playing bowling and enjoying his life. I was informed that his funeral arrangements had been cancelled.

9—MARFAN SYNDROME AND AORTIC ANEURYSM OR DISSECTION

In the early 1960s, a physician published a paper, which stated that President Abraham Lincoln had Marfan syndrome. He certainly had some physical features that made him a suspect: he was taller than most men, had long extremities, and an abnormally shaped chest. This was disputed by other physicians, and at a scientific meeting in October 2001, in Cairo, Egypt, it was concluded that there was not enough evidence to definitely diagnose Lincoln with this disorder.

This is an inherited disorder in 70% of the cases. In 25-30% of Marfan patients, there is no family history of the syndrome. It affects both men and women of any ethnic background. Patients are usually tall, with long, thin arms and legs, and spiderlike fingers called arachnodactyly. Additional physical features include highly arched palate, chest deformity, flat feet, and small lower jaw.

Marfan syndrome is caused by a defect in the building blocks for elastic tissue and organs that contain elastic tissue are particularly affected: the eye shows dislocation of the lens and nearsightedness, the skin is hyperflexible, **and the aorta is weak and fragile and can tear and burst. Patients with Marfan syndrome may develop aortic aneurysms that may rupture or undergo dissection.**

Absolute diagnosis can be made by checking the person's DNA to see if he or she has the defective gene that causes the syndrome.

There is no cure for it, but most people can live a normal life span with good medical care and follow-up.

10—SINUS OF VALSALVA ANEURYSM (SVA)

The sinuses of Valsalva are three outpouchings that originate behind the aortic valve cusps.

The sinus of Valsalva aneurysm (SVA) is due to a congenital weakness of elastic tissue but may also result form atherosclerosis, aortic aneurysms, endocarditis, chest trauma, among other causes.

SVA is estimated to affect one per thousand individuals. They may rupture into a cardiac cavity and cause acute heart failure, or into the pericardial space causing pericardial tamponade. This is accumulation of blood in the pericardial cavity that doesn't allow the heart to contract. SVA usually ruptures between puberty and thirty years of age.

Unruptured SVA usually causes no symptoms and **are generally accidentally detected** by an echocardiogram when it is done for an unrelated condition.

Workup includes MRI (cine magnetic resonance imaging), TEE (trans-esophageal echocardiogram, and 2-D (two-dimensional) echocardiogram. A cardiac catheterization may be necessary.

TREATMENT

A very careful control of the blood pressure is needed. Beta-blockers are useful.

Aggressive surgical correction of an unruptured SVA is often recommended because of the significant mortality that results from its rupture.

11—SPLANCHNIC ARTERY ANEURYSM

In a medical practice, a health care practitioner regularly sees patients who complain of bellyaches. Doctors diagnose gallbladder disease, kidney stone, peptic ulcer, diverticulitis, inflammatory bowel disease, pancreatitis, and other ailments. A frequently unsuspected diagnosis is a splanchnic artery aneurysm.

These focal arterial dilatations develop in **branches of the abdominal aorta that supply blood to the liver, bowel, and spleen.**

From all the aneurysms I described above, the splanchnic artery aneurysms are the ones that are the least popular and recognized by the medical profession. And yet, postmortem studies suggest that these aneurysms are more frequent than abdominal aortic aneurysms. A study by Shabana F. Pasha and associates, published at the *Mayo Clinic Proceedings* warns that it is important to recognize their presence because up to 25% may be complicated by rupture, and the mortality rate after rupture is between 25% and 70% (2007; 82[4]:472-479).

Little is known about the way these vascular abnormalities evolve and their clinical manifestations. Aneurysms of the splenic artery are the most common of the splanchnic aneurysms.

The diagnosis of splanchnic artery aneurysm should be considered in any patient with abdominal pain, a pulsatile mass, or an abdominal bruit. This is a sound heard when a stethoscope is applied by the examiner to the abdomen. Most of these aneurysms, however, give no symptoms and are incidental findings during abdominal surgery done for unrelated reasons or are detected on imaging studies. Treatment is either surgical, or radiology-based interventional procedure becomes a consideration if the aneurysm is greater than 2 cm in diameter, if the patient is pregnant, or if there is demonstrated growth of the aneurysm.

PART 2

ASPHYXIA

We don't appreciate the pleasure of breathing until we lose it.

Asphyxia occurs when there is a severe deficiency of oxygen in the body that results from inability to breathe normally. Poor oxygen concentration in a body tissue is called hypoxia. The brain is very sensitive to it.

Asphyxia is usually but not always accompanied by air hunger. Many mistakenly believe that poor oxygen absorption is responsible for this symptom, but in reality, what mostly triggers the air hunger is the elevated levels of carbon dioxide. Sometimes, victims become hypoxic without being aware of it. Unless action is taken to reverse the process and eliminate the cause of the asphyxia, unconsciousness, brain damage, and death will occur.

Asphyxia is a morbid participant in tortures, capital punishment, suicide, and warfare. Nonfatal asphyxia is also seen in martial arts and combat sports. Erotic sex practices include provoked asphyxiation to heighten sexual pleasure.

12—AIRWAY OBSTRUCTION (CHOKING) IN ADULTS

Dying is never a pleasure, but there are ways and ways of wrestling with this process. Some deaths are painless whereas others can be pretty nasty. Choking due to respiratory tract obstruction by a piece of food is one of them. The victim despairs and perceives the imminence of his or her own demise. This at times can be avoided, and the victim can be saved by a person who knows how to apply a lifesaving maneuver that I described below.

Choking occurs because food goes down the trachea instead of the normal path, the esophagus.

Ways to Avoid It

- Take small bites of food and thoroughly chew it
- Don't laugh or talk while chewing and swallowing
- Excessive booze predisposes to choking
- Do not chew a gum while eating
- Foods tend to stick in the pharynx in the elderly, physically disabled, and helpless.
- Food aspiration (aspiration from gastric contents) can cause a **severe laryngeal spasm** and asphyxia
- Following operations and the removal of the endotracheal tube used during anesthesia, some patients develop critical **laryngeal spasm that closes the glottis and quickly go into pulmonary edema. This is called post-obstruction pulmonary edema (POPE)**
- Those who choke and have full consciousness usually place both hands against the throat. They appear anxious. A person who is unable to speak and only uses hand gestures to communicate needs immediate help
- **Call 911 or ask a bystander to do it right away**
- **If a person is alone and begins to choke, they can perform the Heimlich maneuver on themselves. A clenched fist is placed above the navel, with the other hand on top. Then, the fist should be pushed backward into the stomach with a hard, upward movement. If there's another person, he/she should place the clenched fist above the navel and thrust it backward the way it was just described**

If he or she becomes unconscious and the object has still not been expelled, one must do the following:

- He or she should be positioned flat on his/her back if no obvious injuries are present.
- The jaw should be lifted forward, and a finger should be used to "sweep" the back of the throat and try to remove the foreign object from the throat
- If this is not successful, the "rescuer" should place his/her mouth over the victim's mouth and give two quick deep breaths

- If the windpipe is still blocked, resistance to the breaths will be felt. In this case, up to five abdominal thrusts are given while leaning over the victim
- These motions of providing mouth-to-mouth deep breaths and abdominal thrusts should continue until help arrives

Even when a patient recovers from a serious airway obstruction, it is advisable to be checked by a physician.

Everybody should know how to do the Heimlich maneuver. It is so easy to perform that even your pet can learn to do it. So gather your family in the living room and start practicing it tonight.

13—CARBON MONOXIDE POISONING

Watch for that silent, invisible, odorless, tasteless, treacherous killer.

Carbon monoxide poisoning is responsible for a number of suicidal deaths. In Australia, suicide by young people has attained an alarming rate in recent years, higher than that in the United States and other countries. **The use of motor-vehicle exhaust gas for suicidal purposes has become popular. Authorities are trying to control this problem by limiting the availability of the lethal component carbon monoxide (CO) in motor-vehicle exhaust gas, hoping that the measure will save a few hundred lives per year.**

The choice of CO for suicidal purposes is due to its availability, ease of use, and supposed painless induction. Dr. Jack Kevorkian used to assist terminally ill patients to die using various methods. CO was one of them. He publicly championed a terminal patient's right to die via physician-assisted suicide (for additional information about Dr. Kevorkian and his methods, please see "Euthanasia").

But what about people who do not want to die? Unfortunately, many of them become victims of this gas anyway.

Carbon monoxide is one of the most toxic substances you'll come into contact with in your daily life—in your home, your garage,

your boat, and at work due to defective installations, failure of an appliance, or poor ventilation.

This gas is a byproduct of combustion. Fuels capable of causing carbon monoxide intoxication include propane, natural gas, kerosene, heating oil, wood, and charcoal. So potential sources of carbon monoxide are gas stoves, fireplaces, wood-burning stoves, water heaters, room heaters, furnaces, or any appliance that burns fuel. Carbon monoxide is produced in excess when the fuel doesn't burn cleanly. This is the reason why one needs to do periodic revision of appliances, vehicle, and fireplace.

Hundreds of people die annually from CO poisoning.

Common problems occur during winter when furnaces are turned on and people stay indoors for longer periods. Ventilation is reduced, and the risk of CO poisoning increases. If the car exhaust went bad, a person may get ill while driving the car for some distances, especially if the windows are closed. Smokers are more sensitive to CO poisoning than nonsmokers.

HOW DOES THIS POISON WORK?

It enters the lungs and displaces oxygen from the bloodstream. CO combines with the hemoglobin of the red blood cells and forms carboxyhemoglobin.

Symptoms of CO intoxication include headaches, dizziness, drowsiness, fatigue, shortness of breath, nausea, and vomiting. If you ever experience some of these symptoms when you enter the house or drive your car, and the symptoms disappear after breathing fresh air, suspect that you might have been temporarily intoxicated with carbon monoxide. When exposure to CO is not interrupted, things get worse, and far more disturbing and dangerous: the person becomes unconscious, the heart gets involved in the struggle, and death occurs. The severity of the CO intoxication depends upon the duration of exposure, the size of the area, and the CO concentration.

A common problem is that people fail to associate drowsiness and headaches with CO intoxication. A person who doesn't recognize the situation goes to sleep and may die.

WHO ARE AT A GREATER RISK?

Infants; small children; pets; pregnant women; the unborn baby; cardiac patients; those who suffer from chronic bronchitis, emphysema, and asthma, or have fever, hyperthyroidism, or are alcoholics.

HOW IS THE DIAGNOSIS OF CO INTOXICATION MADE?

By measuring the level of carbon monoxide in the blood. Now remember that carbon monoxide does not stay in the bloodstream long. If your symptoms disappear, the CO levels in the blood may be normal.

PRECAUTIONS TO AVOID CO POISONING

- Suspect it
- Diagnose it
- Evacuate the affected person immediately
- Have your heating system inspected and serviced once a year
- Have your chimney and vents checked regularly
- Never burn charcoal indoors, in the garage or in a tent or van while camping
- Never use a gas range or oven for heating a room
- Never leave a car running in a garage
- Install quality carbon monoxide detectors in your home
- Investigate the source of carbon monoxide and make repairs
- Teach everybody you know what you learned from reading this chapter

IF A PERSON HAS CO POISONING

- Ventilate the area, and if possible, administer oxygen
- If patient is not breathing, perform artificial respiration as taught in cardiopulmonary resuscitation
- Oxygen is the antidote for carbon monoxide. For mild intoxication in healthy people, fresh air may be sufficient. That will help to breath out carbon monoxide. More serious incidents must be treated in the hospital where oxygen is administered, and the heart is monitored. Hyperbaric oxygen may be required in critical cases

CARBON MONOXIDE DETECTORS

*   Look for them in hardware stores
*   Get one that is easily self-tested and easy to reset
*   Do not install it on the ceiling but on a wall where it is easily accessible
*   If it is battery operated, remember to replace the batteries on time
*   If the alarm sounds, ventilate the house immediately
*   Leave the house fast and take your family and pets with you
*   Call your utility company to confirm the CO levels
*   Check the house for the source or sources of this gas

14—CHEST COMPRESSION (COMPRESSIVE ASPHYXIA)

When I was eight years of age, my father took me to a soccer stadium. After the game was over, we tried to get out of that exceedingly crowded place. Thousands rushed to the exit gates. At one point I told my father: "Dad, I can't breathe." My father immediately picked me up and placed me on his shoulders. That was my solution. But then, I feared for his chest compression by the crowd. Fortunately, we made it. That was the last time I went to a soccer stadium.

It's been postulated that a human being can adequately breathe without being able to expand his or her chest but *only* as long as she/he can expand her/his abdomen, allowing for effective diaphragm excursion.

In crowd-related chest-compression death ("riot crush") there is a consistent lack of rib fracture, and it is likely that the cause of death in these cases is abdominal compression—not chest compression. **Be that as it may, fatal crowd accidents have shown that when people have stacked up on each other forming a human pile, the lowest layer is compressed by a weight of about 380 kg (836 lbs).**

A person may become a victim while trying to repair a car using a car jack from below and gets crushed in the thorax when the car jack slips.

Chest compression is sometimes seen in mental health facilities or in individuals under police custody, when a person becomes so violent that the personnel tries a "self-defensive" act. The hold is maintained until help arrives. The victim is exposed to chest compression by the staff member's body weight and arm pressure. If the face is pushed against the coach an airway obstruction may result. The associated neck compression reduces cerebral blood flow.

These three elements, chest compression, face pushed against the coach, and neck compression, represent a lethal combination. In a reported case that ended in death, their application lasted 4-7 minutes.

Other cases of compressive asphyxia are associated with the use of poseys, hogties, bedrails, and choke holds. Asphyxiation of patients by chest compression has resulted from wrapping the arm across the chest and the weight of the staff member on top of the patient while the patient was prone, and after, applying this maneuver for an extended period of time (5-15 minutes).

Smothering or **homicidal asphyxia-suffocation** is the mechanical obstruction of the airway (mouse or nostrils) when these are covered by a hand, a bag, or a pillow. **Overlay** occurs when an adult **accidentally** rolls over an infant who's sleeping in the same bed. Other mechanisms are cave-ins or when a person is buried in sand or grain.

Martial arts chest compression by a technique called leg scissors (also named body scissors), where the legs are wrapped around the opponent's midsection of the thorax and is squeezed, can certainly cause asphyxia and death if done with specific intent.

Compressive asphyxia has been also used as a torture or execution alternative.

Chest compression applied for more than four minutes may result in severe prolonged cerebral hypoxia (lack of oxygen in the brain) and death. **Mental health institutions and police need to follow the specific guidelines of their respective institutions to restrain violent persons in the proper way.**

15—CHOKING, STRANGULATION, AND SUFFOCATION IN CHILDREN

Infants and small children need constant supervision. Many of these deaths by unintentional choking, strangulation, and suffocation can be avoided. A very young child needs your full protection. Bringing up children is a full-time job. You've got to know what they do when they are awake, when they eat, breathe, walk, and sleep. You need to know who sees them, who touches them, who feeds them, and who plays with them.

Airway obstruction is the leading cause of unintentional injury-related death among infants under age one. Oxygen is prevented from reaching the lungs and the brain. This kind of injury occurs when children are unable to breathe normally either because of the following:

a. Food or an object blocks their internal airways **(choking)**
b. Materials cover their external airways and exert pressure on them **(suffocation)**
c. Certain objects are wrapped around their neck **(strangulation)**

Children, and specially under age three, are more vulnerable to airway-obstruction death because they have small airways, don't have enough experience with chewing, and practice the bad habit of putting whatever they find in their mouths.

The majority of childhood chokings, suffocations, and strangulations occur in the home. Risk of choking is prevalent with candies, hot dogs, nuts, grapes, marshmallows, popcorn.

Sixty percent of infant suffocation occurs in the sleeping room or sleeping environment. The incident occurs when the infant's face becomes wedged against or buried in a mattress, pillow, cushion, or when someone sharing the bed rolls over on to him/her. Plastic bags pressed against an infant's mouth and nose may also result in suffocation.

Infants' inability to lift their heads or extricate themselves from tight places puts them at greater risk.

As many as 900 infants died annually in the United States of sudden infant death syndrome (SIDS). They are frequently found on their stomachs with their mouths and noses covered by soft bedding.

Strangulation commonly occurs with drawstrings, ribbons or other decorations, necklaces, pacifier strings, and window blind and drapery cords, when the cord is hanging near the floor or crib.

Symptoms of Airway Obstruction by a Foreign Body: choking or gagging when the object is first inhaled; cough and wheezing when the child breathes; inability to speak; pain in the throat, hoarse voice or/and blueness around the lips.

PREVENTION TIPS

- Place an infant on his/her back on a firm, flat crib mattress that meets national standards. Remove pillows, comforters, toys, and other products from the crib
- Never hang anything on or above a crib with string or ribbon longer than seven inches
- Do not allow children under age six to eat small foods, careful with hot dogs
- Keep safety pins, jewelry, and buttons out of children's reach
- Learn first aid CPR
- Examine toys and search for parts that a child may insert in his/her mouth
- Remove hood and neck drawstrings from all children's outerwear
- Never allow children to wear necklaces, purses, scarves, or clothing with drawstrings
- Tie up all window blind and drapery cords
- Never place a crib near a window
- Ensure that all spaces between the guardrail and bed frame and all spaces in the head and footboards are less than 3.5 in.

TREATMENT AT HOME

- Choking is an emergency and can result in death quickly if not treated promptly. Do not waste time calling your doctor. Call 911 instead
- Call for emergency help. Do not attempt to drive a choking person to a hospital emergency room
- Have other bystanders call the 911 emergency. While waiting for the ambulance, begin first aid immediately
- Do not give the patient anything to drink. Fluids may take up space needed for the passage of air
- If a person starts to choke, is coughing, but is not turning a bluish color, ask, "Are you coughing?" If the person answers you speaking, he or she has a partial airway obstruction. It may be best not to do anything except encourage the person to cough
- A patient who is unable to speak and can only nod the head has a complete airway obstruction and needs emergency help
- Treatment approach at home for a choking person who is turning blue varies with the person's age. In adult or children older than one

year of age, abdominal thrusts (also known as the Heimlich maneuver) should be attempted. This maneuver creates an artificial cough, and sometimes it is forceful enough to expel the foreign body occupying the airway

These quick upper abdominal thrusts force the diaphragm upward very suddenly making the chest cavity smaller. This results in compression of the lungs, which forces the air out, and when successful, the foreign body comes out with it.

HOW TO PERFORM THE HEIMLICH MANEUVER OR ABDOMINAL THRUST

- Lean the person forward slightly and stand behind him or her
- Make a fist with one hand
- Put your arms around the person and grasp your fist with the other hand in the midline, just below the ribs
- Make a quick, hard movement inward and upward. This will help the person to cough up and expel the foreign body. The maneuver should be repeated until the person is able to breathe or loses consciousness

THE HEIMLICH MANEUVER FOR CHOKING INFANTS

- Lay the child down, face up on a firm surface, and kneel or stand at the victim's feet, or hold infant on your lap facing away from you
- Place the middle and index fingers of both your hands below his rib cage and above his navel
- Press into the victim's upper abdomen with a quick upward thrust. Do not squeeze the rib cage. Be very gentle. Repeat until object is eliminated
- Call 911. The infant should be seen immediately even if the rescue effort was successful

Do not

- interfere if the infant is coughing forcefully, has a strong cry, or is breathing adequately
- try to grab and pull out the object if the infant is conscious or perform these steps if the infant stops breathing for other reasons, such as asthma, or a blow to the head

16—LARYNGEAL SPASM

This condition is an unpredictable, uncontrolled, involuntary contraction (spasm) of the larynx (voice box). It typically lasts for 30-60 seconds and causes a partial blocking of breathing while breathing out remains unaffected.

Persons who undergo surgery and need general anesthesia must be inserted a tube in the trachea to assist the respiratory function during the operation (endotracheal intubation). The tube is removed after surgery immediately, hours, or days following the operation depending upon each particular situation. After removal of the endotracheal tube, the patient must be watched carefully since severe laryngeal spasm may develop. This may also occur when the endotracheal tube **is not** removed, and the larynx detects the entry of water or other substances. It produces a high-pitched screamlike sound. The affected person may be awake or asleep.

Laryngeal spasm is frequently seen in people who have silent esophageal reflux.

In the operating room, it is treated by hyperextending the patient's head and providing mechanical ventilation with 100% oxygen. If the spasm is significant, the patient needs to be inserted the endotracheal tube again. If introduction of an endotracheal tube is not possible, the larynx must be opened through a surgical incision in the anterior neck to create an airway.

In regular medical practice, when laryngeal spasms are due to acid reflux going from the stomach into the esophagus, the patient should be reassured and treated with antireflux medications.

17—POSITIONAL ASPHYXIA

Restraining a person with the face down and pressing his/her thorax or holding an individual around the neck may be lethal.

It is also called postural asphyxia and occurs when a person's body position prevents her/him from breathing adequately. Some people may die when they are subjected to excessive and/or inadequate restraint techniques used by police, prison officers, and health care personnel.

Restraining a person in a face-down position is likely to cause greater restriction of breathing than restraining a person face up.

Law enforcement officers and health care personnel are currently taught to avoid restraining people with the face down or to do so for a very short period of time.

If the individual subjected to this kind of treatment suffers from cardiopulmonary disease, is severely obese, or is under the influence of alcohol and/or drugs, is placed with the face down or any type of restraint is held around the neck, there is an increase probability of death.

18—SEX AND EROTIC ASPHYXIA

Individuals who seek sexual pleasure enhancement—erotic excitement and orgasms—by intentionally inducing asphyxiation methods suffer from a mental disorder known as **hypoxyphilia or erotic asphyxiation**. It is done as a form of masturbation (autoerotic asphyxiation) or with a partner. **This activity is very dangerous and may end in death.**

The usual techniques are the following:

- A plastic bag is applied over the head
- Self-strangulation by applying a ligature (scarfing) around the neck

In 2004, the right-wing National Front party member Kristian Etchells died during a sex act of this kind. On March 28, 2007, the *New York Times* had a front-page story on a teenager who had suffered a heart attack and spent three days in a coma after hanging himself for a "rush."

Some of those involved with these practices are not fully aware about the possible dreadful consequences of erotic asphyxiation. They think they're having fun. That is, until their cyanotic, blue, and inert faces prove how wrong they were.

This abnormal human behavior is not new. Historically, the practice dates back to the 1600s. Men who were executed by hanging were noted to develop an erection and sometimes ejaculation during the execution. Sometimes, the erection remained after dying.

PART 3

CENTRAL NERVOUS SYSTEM DISORDERS

19—AGITATED DELIRIUM—ACUTE EXCITED STATES

Unless you've seen a person suffering this crisis, you can't imagine what he/she and those involved in his/her care go through. It's a very impressive scene, and if you are part of the team to control this reaction, you've got to be prepared for it and get ready for action. And it isn't a good sight. I can assure you that!

Agitated delirium (AD) is an acute onset of bizarre and violent behavior associated with hyperactivity, accompanied by combativeness, hyperactivity, unexpected display of great physical strength, senseless shouting, hallucinations, and high fever (hyperthermia).

The underlying causes of this disorder include manic-depressive psychosis, chronic schizophrenia, cocaine intoxication, alcohol withdrawal, head trauma, and intoxication with sympathomimetics or anticholinergics.

Sympathomimetic drugs are cathecolamines or analogs of cathecolamines that can produce excessive cardiac stimulation and cardiac arrhythmias. **Anticholinergics** are substances that block the neurotransmitter acetylcholine and are used to treat gastrointestinal disorders (gastritis, diverticulitis, colitis), respiratory disorders (asthma), Parkinson's disease, and others.

Emergency medical services (EMS) or police are frequently the first to face these cases. Since restraining efforts are unavoidable, caution is warranted in exercising them. Patients need to be tackled and physically restrained. Chemical restraint is also important (e.g., with haloperidol).

Some of these patients go into respiratory or cardiac arrest and cannot be resuscitated.

I participated in the acute care of a number of patients suffering from agitated delirium when I was a medical resident in the mid-1960s. We had a ward of alcoholic and psychotic patients. Alcohol withdrawal reactions were common. During the night shift, I was responsible for these patients, and I was assisted by a couple of interns, nurses, and security personnel. Some of them became violent, and we were all afraid of being hurt or even killed. We had to act quickly to prevent loss of human life or severe injuries. The patient was agitated and so was every person in the room. The patient was cursing, insulting, and attacking anybody on sight. What did I do? I'll tell you what I did: I ordered "Get the f—net fast!'" This was a huge net we were authorized to use as the last resort to restrain violent patients, that is, if other less dramatic methods had failed. In a few seconds the net was thrown over the patient, and then four very strong men held him, and a nurse managed to inject a sedative that was provided through one of the net's holes.

This experience was kind of pathetic. The patient was trapped inside the net and acted like a tiger trying to come out of it. The intervention, however, was justified, and patients were safely treated without serious complications.

WHY DO PATIENTS WITH AGITATED DELIRIUM DIE?

These are the probable mechanisms of sudden death in patients with AD.

- *Positional asphyxia.* Some patients die shortly after they were placed in physical restraints in a prone position, particularly after being hog-tied. This consists of placing the subject prone and binding wrists and ankles together behind the back. The U.S. Department of Justice has issued a guidance statement cautioning against the use of hog-tying. (Please also see section **16 "Positional Asphyxia."**)
- *Metabolic acidosis.* The stress these patients go through may cause cardiovascular collapse that also usually occurs following exertion in a restrained position. This results in accumulation of toxic acids

and a condition termed metabolic acidosis that can lead to cardiac arrest

- *Rhabdomyolysis.* This muscular tissue necrosis (destruction) is observed in chronic cocaine users. This condition is associated with bizarre and agitated behavior. Those who have concomitant high fever (hyperthermia) are even more prone to develop severe cardiac arrhythmias

- *Catecholamine-induced sudden death.* The role of catecholamines and stress has been studied in cases of sudden death. Stress is known to increase mortality of preexisting heart disease. Patients with AD appear to be specially sensitive to catecholamines

HOW TO APPROACH THESE PATIENTS

- Measures must be taken to assure the safety of the patient and the medical team dealing with this crisis. Not restraining the patient leads to chaos, and restraining the patient too roughly may provoke his/her cardiac or respiratory arrest
- The mere presence of police officials may aggravate the patient's agitation
- The patient should not be restrained in a prone position if at all possible
- Maintaining him or her in a supine or lateral position may help minimize the risk of a compromised airway
- Combativeness is best treated with an injection of a benzodiazepine for sedation
- Patients with AD, especially those who have a history of cocaine use or psychosis, are at risk for sudden death
- Respiratory and cardiac function should be monitored. Emergency medical personnel should be aware of the possible complications of AD and be prepared to address them

20—BRAIN INJURIES IN GENERAL AND IN SPORTS

A traumatic brain injury usually results from a sudden, violent blow to the head. This shakes the brain and makes it collide with the inside of the skull. The bones of the skull are difficult to break. Brain injury without a fractured skull is known as closed—head injury. **Although sports injuries contribute to fatalities infrequently, the leading cause of death from sports-related injuries is traumatic brain injury (TBI).**

Sports and recreational activities contribute to about 21% of all traumatic brain injuries among American children and adolescents. The severity of the brain injury varies according to the affected part of the brain and the extent of the damage.

Approximately 1.4 million Americans suffer a traumatic brain injury **(TBI)** each year. **Three hundred thousand of these injuries are sports related**. More than 75% of the TBI are mild. **One point to keep in mind though is that minor head injuries can cause long-term problems.**

These are the sports or recreational activities that contribute to the highest numbers of estimated head injuries treated in U.S. hospital emergency rooms:

- Cycling
- Powered recreational vehicles, dune buggies
- Football
- Basketball
- Baseball and softball (when batting)
- Water sports (diving, scuba diving, surfing, swimming, water polo, water skiing)
- Skateboards/scooters
- Soccer
- Winter sports (skiing, sledding, snowboarding, snowmobiling)
- Horseback riding
- Health club exercise, weight lifting
- Golf
- Trampolines
- Gymnastics/dance/cheerleading
- Hockey
- Balls sports (unspecified)
- Skating (in line, roller, roller hockey)
- Wrestling
- Boxing
- Fishing
- Ice skating

Injuries that do not appear too serious may indeed be fatal.

Brain injuries act on two stages: (1) the actual injury, and (2) the brain swelling. When brain swells up, the intracranial pressure increases, and unless this is corrected, brain damage occurs.

The most frequent causes of head injuries are the following:

- Car accidents (passenger and pedestrian)
- Biclycle/motorcycle accidents
- Falls (especially children and the elderly)
- Sports
- Acts of violence/assault

Types and Symptoms of Head Injuries

Most head injuries are preventable. Most head injuries do not result in permanent brain damage.

These are some of the most common types:

- Loss of consciousness
- Concussion: temporary mental confusion
- Brain contusion: bruise in the brain causing swelling
- Skull fracture
- Hematoma: clot collection inside the brain

Motor Vehicle Accidents and Head Injuries

Fifty thousand children are hit by a car each year. Quite frequently, the resulting head injuries are serious. Over 50% of all head injuries in the United States involve car accidents.

Seat belts and air bags are the best methods of prevention when riding in the car. It is estimated that seat belts have saved about 55,000 fatalities in the past decade.

For preventive measures for bicycle, motorcycle accidents and falls, please see "Accidents."

BRAIN INJURY IN SPORTS

The guidelines provided below are those of the Brain Injury Resource Center.

212 Pioneer Bldg
Seattle, WA 98104-2221
brain@headinjury.com
http://www.headinjury.com

There is an increased risk in repeat injuries. Mild brain injuries occurring over an extended period (i.e., months or years) can result in cumulative neurological and cognitive deficits, but repeated mild brain injuries occurring within a short period of time (i.e., hours, days, weeks) can be catastrophic or fatal. The latter phenomenon termed "second impact syndrome" has been increasingly recognized since it was first identified in 1984.

A typical, expected sequence of events would occur as follows: a football player is tackled and struck his head on the ground. A while later he complains of a headache. Plays again in the third quarter and receives several routine blows to his helmet. He collapses and is taken to a hospital and is pronounced dead in four days. The autopsy reveals brain swelling.

The second impact syndrome is not yet widely recognized, namely the mild, repetitive blows to the head sustained during a short period of time may cause brain swelling, which is responsible for the fatal outcome. After several concussions, it takes less of a blow to cause the injury.

It is thought that once a person suffers a concussion, he/she is as much as four times more likely to sustain a second one.

Concussion is the head-trauma-induced alteration in mental status that may or may not involve loss of consciousness. Concussions are graded in three categories.

Grade 1 Concussion
Symptoms: transient confusion, no loss of consciousness
Duration: less than fifteen minutes
Management: The athlete should be removed from sports activity, examined immediately and at five-minute intervals. He or she is only allowed to return that day to sports activity only if post-concussive symptoms resolve within fifteen minutes. Any athlete who suffers a second grade 1 concussion on the same day should be removed from sports activity until no complaint is voiced for one week.

Grade 2 Concussion
Symptoms: transient confusion, no loss of consciousness
Duration: more than fifteen minutes
Management: The athlete should be removed from sports activity, examined immediately and frequently to evaluate his or her symptoms. If these persist longer than one week, more in-depth evaluation is required. If the athlete is asymptomatic for one week, he/she may return to sports activity a week later.

Any athlete who incurs a grade 2 concussion subsequent to a grade 1 concussion on the same day should be removed from sports activity until asymptomatic for two weeks.

Grade 3 Concussion
Symptom: **loss of consciousness**
Duration: **either for a few seconds (brief) or for minutes or longer (prolonged)**
Management: The athlete is removed from sports activity for one full week without symptoms if the loss of consciousness is brief, or two full weeks without symptoms if the loss of consciousness is prolonged. If still unconscious, or if abnormal neurological signs are present at the time of initial evaluation, the athlete should be transported by ambulance to the nearest hospital emergency room. An athlete who suffers a second grade 3 concussion should be removed from sports activity until asymptomatic for one month.

Any athlete with an abnormality on computed tomography, magnetic resonance imaging, or brain scan consistent with brain swelling, contusion, or any other intracranial abnormality should be removed from sports activities for the season and discouraged from any participation in the future with any kind of contact sports.

HEAD INJURIES IN SOCCER

Soccer injuries are more frequent and more serious than what soccer fans are generally aware of.

In 1999, the team physician for McGill's football and soccer teams realized he was seeing more head injuries in soccer players than in football players. Dr. Scott Delaney noticed that some soccer players were lost for the entire season. Many missed weeks of school unable to keep up with their studies in more advanced fields.

The America Youth Soccer Association (AYSA) represents almost 700,000 players. Members proposed a rule that would ban heading in practices and games for all players under the age of ten. The proposal was narrowly defeated.

Some studies have shown that a surprisingly high percentage of soccer players have neuropsychological deficiencies of attention, concentration, memory, and judgment. These results not only from heading but player collisions and running into goal posts. Children are more susceptible to these injuries because their skulls are thinner and offer less protection to the brain. In addition, their necks are weaker and don't absorb or dissipate forces applied to the head. Dr. Delaney recommended the use of helmet, not similar to the football helmet but one modeled on the old-style leather football helmet.

BOXING

A boxer's fist produces a force that is equivalent to being hit with a thirteen-pound bowling ball traveling twenty miles per hour.

A significant number of boxers have speech difficulties, unsteadiness, memory loss, and abnormal behavior. It is estimated that 15-40% of ex-boxers have symptoms of chronic brain injury. Recent studies have shown that most professional boxers (even those without symptoms) have some degree of brain damage.

CYCLING

Every year, there are 500,000 visits to U.S. hospitals emergency rooms due to bicycle—related injuries. Without proper protection, a fall of as little as two feet can result in traumatic brain injury. Some children do not use the helmet properly (it fits improperly, or they just don't use it).

FOOTBALL

There were forty-four head injury-related deaths from 1995 to 2004.

Conclusion: Many traumatic brain injuries are preventable. Depending upon the sport you or your children practice, use protective equipment when needed and take other precautions that deal with the dynamics of each particular sport activity.

I suggest you to obtain additional information on how to enjoy your favorite sport without getting killed or maimed in the process.

FOR ADDITIONAL INFORMATION

Brain Trauma Foundation (BTF), BTFLearning.org

21—THE "BROKEN HEART" SYNDROME

An intense emotion, such as the sudden, unexpected death of a loved one can trigger sudden heart failure. The picture is different from a classical heart attack and has been studied by cardiologists at John Hopkins University (Ilan Wittstein, MD).

This has been called **stress cardiomyopathy** commonly known as the **broken heart syndrome** and results from the cumulative effect of an adrenaline surge that has been present for several days of intense grief.

Some of those affected by this condition produce symptoms similar to those of an acute heart attack or myocardial infarction, including chest pains, shortness of breath, and heart failure with fluid accumulation in the lungs. Close observation, however, establishes the correct diagnosis. The patient did not have an acute myocardial infarction. Instead, she or he suffered from the broken heart syndrome.

Coronary angiograms typically show no blockage of coronary arteries. The congestive heart failure is reversible, and patient's heart muscle strength returns to normal. Those who suffer an acute myocardial infarction are left with a scar and some contractility disorder of the left ventricle.

In the "broken heart" syndrome, there is massive elevation of catecholamines such as metanephrine and normetanephrine and other stress-related proteins such as neuropeptide Y, brain natriuretic peptide, and serotonin. Heart biopsies showed an injury pattern of the myocardial cells consistent with a high catecholamine state. That is different from a myocardial infarction where the heart muscle damage results from a blocked coronary artery.

The "broken heart" syndrome is not as frequently diagnosed as it deserves to be. Physicians need to be more aware about its existence and recognize its unique clinical features.

22—ENCEPHALITIS

This disease is caused by a large number of viruses. In the United States, there are approximately 20,000 cases reported per year. The disorder has some features seen in cases of meningitis. Its distinction from meningitis is that in addition to the meninges, the membranes that cover the brain, encephalitis also directly affects the brain tissue.

A patient suffering from encephalitis is not mentally alert. There's confusion, disorientation, hallucinations, agitation, behavioral changes, and frequently has slurring of the speech (dysphasia) and inability to move either the right or the left upper and lower extremities.

The diagnosis requires spinal fluid examination, which is done by lumbar (lower spine) puncture. This should never be done without confirming the presence of cerebral edema or brain herniation by MRI (MRI is preferred over CT scan in cases of encephalitis). If a lumbar puncture is done under the mentioned conditions, it may result in sudden death. There are many diseases of the brain that can mimic encephalitis and require expertise to know the difference. Although viral encephalitis is not usually treated with antibiotics, it is important to rule out HSV infection (herpes simplex virus) because there are antiviral drugs that can provide specific therapy.

The outlook of encephalitis in part depends on the offending virus. Some encephalitis are quite benign, and patients recover without sequelae. Others resolved with cerebral or neurological deficits, and others are fatal. For instance, in the case of Eastern equine encephalitis virus infection, nearly 80% of survivors are left with neurological damage, whereas Californian or Venezuelan equine encephalitis rarely caused any kind of permanent neurological damage.

23—MENINGITIS

Meningitis is a serious infection of the membranes that cover the brain. It may be caused by numerous viruses and bacteria. Bacterial meningitis is most common in the winter and is more severe than viral meningitis, particularly in infants and the elderly. I remember the patients screaming their terrible headaches. They also had rigid neck, fever, and altered mental status. The typical neck rigidity seen in adults may be absent in infants. Before antibiotics were used, bacterial meningitis was fatal in 70% or more of cases. With antibiotic treatment, the incidence of fatal outcomes dropped to 5-15%.

The majority of bacterial cases are caused by the *Haemophilus influenzae, Neisseria meningitides, or Streptococcus pneumoniae.* Meningococcal meningitis primarily affects young children whereas pneumococcal meningitis generally strikes infants, the elderly, and individuals debilitated by a number of chronic medical conditions.

The most important test to diagnose meningitis is the examination of the cerebrospinal fluid, which is obtained by introducing a needle in the lower part of the spine. There are situations, though, when this test is risky and should not be performed. **If there is a cerebral mass or elevated intracranial pressure, a lumbar puncture is contraindicated because of the possibility of fatal brain herniation. A CT or MRI scan prior to the lumbar puncture will help rule out this possibility.**

PREVENTION

Immunization. Vaccinations exist against *Haemophilus influenzae,* type A and C *Neisseria meningitides.* Vaccines against type B *Neisseria meningitides* are much harder to produce.

Vaccination against *Streptococcus pneumoniae* is recommended for all people sixty-five years of age or older. Mump vaccination has led to a great decline in mumps-virus-associated meningitis.

HYGIENE MEASURES

Transmission of viral and bacterial meningitis can be prevented by raising the level of hygiene among persons at risk of infection. Wash hands with soap and clean under the fingernails. Use a paper towel or your own towel.

Cover nose and mouth when sneezing. Do not share straws, cups, glasses, cigarettes, or eating utensils. Don't kiss an infant on the mouth.

For meningococcal meningitis, those who had contact with a person suffering from this disease are recommended to receive a preventive antibiotic, often rifampin. This drug kills bacteria living in nose and throat secretions. Same drug may be recommended for prevention of *Haemophilus influenzae* meningitis contacts.

TREATMENT

Bacterial meningitis must be treated with antibiotics. The suspicion of the disease is an immediate indication to get to a hospital emergency department **fast.**

24—PSYCHIC STRESS AND EMOTIONAL REACTION

There is considerable evidence associating acute myocardial infarctions with psychic and environmental stress. The mechanism is increased because of production of catecholamines resulting from stimulation of the sympathetic system, which leads to increased blood pressure, rapid heart rate, augmenting of cardiac contractility, activation of platelets, which increase the propensity for clot formation. The combined action of all these forces on an artery's atherosclerotic plaque may lead to its rupture (plaque rupture), and this in turn, causes the formation of a clot that blocks a coronary artery. This results in an acute (at times fatal) myocardial infarction or a deadly arrhythmia due to an excess of circulating adrenaline or a spasm of a coronary artery that produces ventricular fibrillation.

Anger and distressing life events have been noted to precede for several months the development of an acute myocardial infarction. A cerebral hemorrhage may also be the result of intense aggravation. Hypertensive patients who are also excessive consumers of alcohol are particularly prone to this complication.

The signs of stress are familiar and troubling: anger, anxiety, sleeplessness.

The late eminent cardiologist, Dr. Robert S. Eliot, addressed the issue of stress and related deaths in his book *Is It Worth Dying For?* (Bantam Books, 1987). It is an inspiring work. Although it was published twenty years ago, its principles and conclusions continue to have up to date value. "Modern stress is due in part, to modern lifestyles, and our circuits are overloaded," he stated. As a cardiologist consultant at NASA, he observed the sudden demise of highly paid employees (physicists, scientists, engineers) who had lost their jobs due to budgetary problems and limitations at the space center. In autopsy studies, he saw the effects of high levels of adrenaline and other stress chemicals: these had led to the "literal rupture of heart muscle fibers."

HOW TO REDUCE STRESS

- Accept the fact that sometimes it's better to be alone than with the wrong friend, spouse, or lover
- Aim for flexibility in your commitments
- Allow yourself to express negative feelings
- Consider changing an unfulfilling or aggravating job to a more gratifying one
- Cultivate very good friendships. If you lose a good friend, try to find another one
- Do only one thing at a time
- Don't be a perfectionist
- Don't eat your heart out with hostility and anger. Focus on positive thoughts
- Don't fret about things you cannot change
- Don't try to control other people's behavior
- Finds ways to minimize the pressure of schedules and deadlines
- Find more time to do what you want
- Improve personal relationships
- Take breaks at your job a couple of times a day—and relax
- Try to turn negative feelings into positive ones

Other methods to deal with stress include physical exercise, yoga, meditation, deep breathing, a healthier lifestyle, religious faith, biofeedback, mental relaxation, and a good psychotherapist.

25—SEIZURES

A seizure is always worrisome, and besides urgent management, it requires the proper identification of its cause. **Avoidance of cardio-respiratory arrest that can be fatal is crucial.**

It isn't always medically easy to immediately know why a person is suffering a seizure. There are various precipitating factors, and the sooner the culprit is found, the better are the chances for the victim's recovery.

The person's age helps to suspect the possible cause of the seizure attack.

Infant (up to 2 years of age)

- Perinatal insufficient cerebral oxygenation (hypoxia)
- Intracranial birth injury
- Acute infection
- Hypoglycemia, hypomagnesemia, hypocalcemia, pyridoxine deficiency
- Congenital malformation
- Genetic disorders

Child (2-12)

- Unknown
- Acute infection
- Trauma
- High fever

Adolescent (12-18)

- Trauma
- Alcohol or drug withdrawal
- Cerebral arterial-venous malformation

Young adult (18-35)

- Trauma
- Alcoholism
- Brain tumor

Older adult (> 35)

- Brain tumor
- Cerebrovascular disease
- Uremia (advanced renal insufficiency)
- Hypoglycemia
- Liver failure

- Electrolyte abnormality
- Alcoholism

Note: Epilepsy is a convulsive disorder produced by abnormalities in the electrical activity of the brain that causes paroxysmal attacks. These are estimated to occur in 0.5-2% of the U.S. population and can occur at any age.

MEDICAL APPROACH TO A SEIZURE DISORDER

Initial emergency evaluation is directed toward ensuring adequate ventilation and stopping the seizure. The health care practitioner may obtain useful information from a friend or relative, the physical examination and some lab tests.

Immediate attention must provide adequate respiratory support and proper ventilation, circulatory support, protection of the tongue (with a soft object, large enough not to be swallowed, between the clenched teeth), protection of the head, and then secure an intravenous line. A bolus of 50% glucose is given even if hypoglycemia is not suspected, and this alone may stop the seizures. Whether the seizure disorder is due to epilepsy or any other disturbance, **the specific cause of the seizure must be found and treated accordingly.** Proper management may avoid a fatal complication.

26—STROKE

Essentially, there are two types of strokes: one kind is caused by the **blockage** of a cerebral artery resulting from either an atherosclerotic plaque that forms a clot called thrombus (cerebral thrombosis), or a traveling clot from an aortic or carotid atherosclerotic plaque, or the left atrium, left ventricle, or mitral valve (cerebral embolism). This is called **ischemic stroke. The resulting brain damage is called cerebral infarction.**

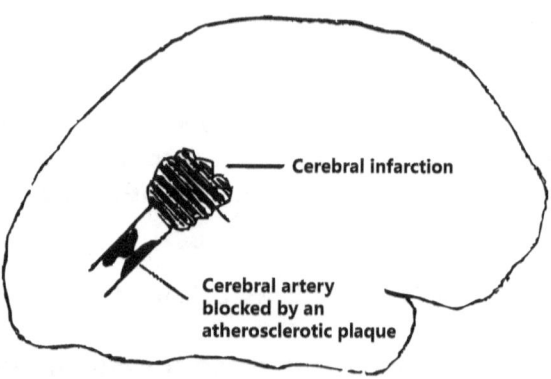

Ischemic stroke-Cerebral infarction

Figure 5

The other mechanism of stroke is **rupture** of a cerebral artery. This is called **hemorrhagic stroke** or **intracerebral hemorrhage (ICH).** Some ICH are small and cause mild neurological damage. However, at times the hemorrhage is massive and may be fatal fast.

Stroke by cerebral thrombosis (or cerebral artery blockage) causes damage depending upon the size and location of the affected area of the brain: paralysis of the upper and lower extremities, visual deficits, speech impairment, mental confusion and or a number of mental function abnormalities, soft palate paralysis and inability to swallow, and other deficits.

Young persons suffer strokes less commonly than older persons, but their strokes are more likely to be hemorrhagic than ischemic strokes.

A stroke caused by a cerebral hemorrhage is always a medical emergency. It causes 10-15% of all strokes. **It usually results from hypertension, eclampsia (also called toxemia of pregnancy), a ruptured cerebral aneurysm, arterio-venous malformations (AVM), or abuse of certain drugs. The combination of hypertension and alcoholism greatly predisposes to cerebral hemorrhage.**

At times, a cerebral hemorrhage is a complication of a clot-dissolving drug used to open up an artery blocked by a clot. In other words, in such cases, the treatment of an ischemic stroke is complicated by a hemorrhagic stroke.

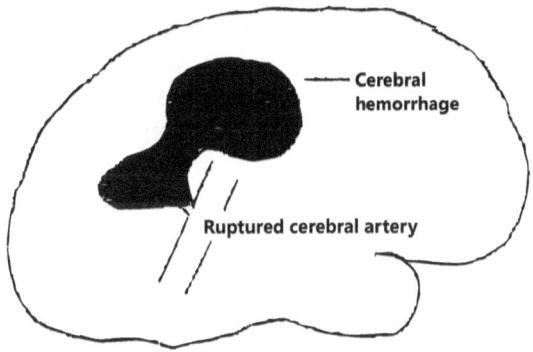

Hemorrhagic stroke-Cerebral hemorrhage

Figure 6

For reasons that are not clearly understood, pregnancy increases hemorrhagic stroke risk, and women who have just given birth are more than twenty-eight times more likely to suffer a hemorrhagic stroke than the average individual.

A cerebral hemorrhage typically presents with sudden, severe headache; stiff neck; pain in the face, between the eyes; visual disturbances; vomiting; and altered consciousness.

Immediate neurosurgical evaluation is mandatory. Cerebral angiography determines the precise cause and site of the bleeding. This is important because in certain cases of ICH, when a ruptured cerebral aneurysm is identified, emergency surgery to "clip" the aneurysm off from the normal brain blood circulation is carried out.

Nimodipine is a drug that has been shown to reduce the incidence of vasospasm, a worrisome complication frequently seen with this type of stroke.

Subarachnoid hemorrhage (SAH) is bleeding into the subarachnoid space surrounding the brain in between the arachnoid membrane and the pia mater. It may arise due to trauma, or spontaneously, most often due to rupture of a cerebral aneurysm. It is a particularly dangerous type of stroke. SAH causes 5% of all strokes, and 10-15% of patients die before arriving to the hospital. The average survival is 50%.

The classic presentation is an unbearable headache that develops in seconds to minutes. Other features include vomiting, seizures, confusion, coma. **This condition must be recognized quickly, and emergent neurosurgical consultation is mandatory**. For more details on diagnosis and treatment, **please see section 5 "Cerebral Aneurysm."**

27—SUICIDE

Prompt recognition of major depression prevents suicide. Sometimes, symptoms of severe depression elude timely diagnosis and treatment, and a disastrous outcome results. In a period of a few years, three physicians working in my community committed suicide. They all made rounds in the hospital shortly before their tragic decisions, said "Hello, Ed," as usual, and visited their patients, as usual. Their souls were tormented, but they kept that deep anguish to themselves. That of course, is not good.

An elderly deaf-mute patient of mine who was hospitalized for severe depression refused to drink or eat. He just wanted to die. He was given intravenous fluids, which he violently pulled out. A gastric feeding tube was provided, and he did the same. The consulting psychiatrist ended his report with these words: "If this patient so badly wants to die, he will!" It just took him a couple of more days to get what he wanted.

**

Ana was seventy years of age and attempted suicide a couple of times with sedatives but was successfully treated. I refrained from prescribing her anything that would even remotely have a sedative action and asked the psychiatrist and other specialists taking care of her to do the same. What did she do? She swallowed a full bottle containing one hundred tablets of a drug to treat her diabetes. She got her wish!

Depression and suicide are closely related.

It is estimated that approximately 90% of those who commit suicide had an existing mental illness or substance abuse problem at the time of their death.

Depression may present as the following:

In Children

- School phobia or school avoidance, head banging, or self-biting
- Harming animals
- Unusual disobedience
- Low self-esteem
- Eating or sleeping problems
- Bedwetting, constipation or diarrhea
- Panic attacks
- Disorganized speech
- Headaches, or pain in various areas of the body
- Suicidal talk or attempts

In Adolescents

- Eating disorder (anorexia or bulimia)
- Drug or alcohol abuse
- Sexual promiscuity
- Carelessness while walking across busy streets or bridges
- Physical or sexual assaults against others
- Obnoxious behavior
- Social isolation
- Running away
- Deficient personal appearance and hygiene
- Immoral acts
- Uncontrollable anger, irritability, constant unhappiness
- Lack of energy, sluggishness
- Excessive fears
- Suicidal thoughts or attempts

In Adults

- Persistent sadness
- Hopelessness
- Pessimistic and guilty
- Substance abuse
- Loss of interest in ordinary activities, including sex
- Eating and/or sleeping disturbances
- Irritability, excessive crying, panic attacks
- Persistent physical complaints, pains in different areas of the body

- Difficulties in concentrating—memory deficits
- Suicidal thoughts or attempts
- Talks about suicide: "I have no interest in living." "I'd like to kill myself."
- Saying good-byes to people one cares about
- Giving things away
- Refusal to follow medical instructions

Depression can be treated successfully in about 90% of the patients with medications and psychotherapy. Some depressions in the elderly may respond to ECT (electroconvulsive therapy). This treatment is usually reserved for cases of severe depression when a rapid improvement is indicated.

WHERE TO GET HELP

- Your family health care practitioner
- Mental health professionals, psychiatrists, psychologists, family therapists, and social workers
- Community mental health centers
- Hospitals
- University medical schools

SUICIDAL IDEAS: WHAT TO DO

If you have thoughts of suicide, do the following:

- Dial 911.
- Dial 1-800-273-TALK.
- Go to a hospital emergency room immediately.
- Keep away from things that might hurt you.
- Have faith and confidence that your condition has very good chances of improving dramatically with psychotherapy and medications.
- **The most important step is to talk to someone. Don't try to cope with this problem alone. Seek help *now*! If you feel suicidal, talk about your feelings immediately!**

If you don't have medical insurance, do the following:

- Go to the nearest hospital emergency room.

- Look in the local yellow pages under "Mental Health" and/or "Suicide Prevention" and call the listed phone lines. Some counseling centers can accommodate you with no fee scale or a sliding fee scale.
- Some pharmaceutical companies have "free medication programs" for those who qualify. Visit the National Alliance for the Mentally Ill Web site at *www.nami.org* for additional information.

EMERGENCY NUMBERS

If you are in crisis, call 911.

The yellow pages usually list the local suicide prevention hotline or crisis center. The Trevor Project (866-488-7386) is aimed at gay and youth who are in trouble. They have a toll-free suicide prevention hotline. Consultations are handled by highly trained professional. These are free and confidential.

Girls and Boys Town crisis line (twenty-four hours a day, every day)	800-448-3000
Alcohol @ Drug Abuse hotline	800-454-8966
Children of the Night	800-551-1300
National Alcohol @ Drug Abuse hotline	800-252-6465
National Hopeline Network Crisis hotline	800-442-4673
National Network of Runaway Youth Services	202-783-7949

PART 4

DRUGS

28—DRUG OVERDOSE

This happens when you consume more drugs than your body is able to tolerate. An overdose is a serious event. It can be dangerous and leads to unconsciousness and death. People who want to get "high" with drugs walk on a tightrope. Sometimes, the distance between being "high" and being "dead" is barely perceptible.

Those who take heroin or other drugs frequently make an additional mistake: they combine these drugs with alcohol. This accelerates the transition to a lethal outcome.

Depressants slow you down and increase the risk of fainting or stopping of breathing. Stimulants speed you up and heighten the risks of seizures or heart attacks.

Taking any of these drugs increases the risk of death. Drug overdose may not kill you fast. Sometimes, organs are damaged, and there is kidney or liver failure that occasionally ends in dialysis or liver transplantation. Severe impairment of the respiratory and circulatory systems is something that you may need to reckon with. A real mess!

Drugs are classified as either of the following:

- **Prescription drugs** (Valium, morphine, benzodiazepines [sleeping medications])
- **Nonprescription drugs**: these can be purchased over the counter to deal with headaches, cough, diarrhea, constipation, headaches, and

a number of other common conditions. Alcohol and the nicotine of cigarettes also enter into this category

- **Illicit drugs:** these are drugs that are imported, grown, or manufactured illegally. They are from dangerous to lethal and usually cause dependence or addiction (heroin, cocaine, amphetamines, ecstasy, LSD)

A drug overdose may result from the following:

- Intention to inflict self-damage (suicide attempt)
- Illicit drug consumption with or without additional use of alcohol
- Accidental administration
- Medical error and excessive doses of a medication

Symptoms of overdose vary:

- Sleepiness on antiepileptics, hypoglycemia on insulin
- Liver failure in Tylenol intoxication or metabolic acidosis with aspirin
- Confusion, vertigo, nausea, vomiting, delirium, seizures

Diagnosis is easy when the ingested drug is identified and difficult if the patient doesn't know or refuses to state what drug he or she ingested. **Treatment** is supportive in most cases. Sometimes it is specific: naloxone in opiods and flumazenil in benzodiazepines. The effect of the offending drug is reversed. **Immediate action** may prevent a death that would occur in a few hours.

DEPRESSANTS

- Opiates (morphine, heroin, methadone)
- Alcohol
- Benzodiazepines

Signs of overdose: slow, shallow breathing; blue fingernails and lips; cold, pale skin; snoring or gargling noises; unresponsiveness

WHAT TO DO

If Someone Suffers a Reaction after Taking a Drug and Gets Panicky

- Be calm and reassuring
- Explain that the feeling will pass
- Move the person to a room where there are no bright lights, noisy music, or is not crowded
- If the person is hyperventilating, encourage him or her to relax and take a long, slow, deep breath

If Someone Gets Drowsy

This happens with alcohol, sedatives, heroin, and solvents

- Dial 911 and call an ambulance immediately
- Place them in the recovery position
- Never give them coffee to rouse them. The offending drug might work faster

If the Victim is Unresponsive

- See if she or he is breathing
- If breathing and pulse are not detected, start CPR (cardiopulmonary resuscitation). If these signs are present, roll the person on his/her side into the recovery position
- Call an ambulance. Ideally, one person implements the previous recommendations and another calls 911

STIMULANTS

- Amphetamines
- Cocaine

Signs of overdose: rapid heartbeat, confusion, psychosis, seizures, muscle cramps, unresponsiveness, and possibly cardiac arrest

WHAT TO DO

First aid: Stay with the person and help him/her to remain calm. Move the victim to a quiet area. If unconscious, place the patient in the recovery position and call an ambulance.

PREVENTION

- Never mix depressant drugs with alcohol, barbiturates, benzodiazepines, and opiates
- Always start with a low dose to test effect of the drug and your tolerance to it
- Be careful when taking a depressant drug after a period of abstinence as your tolerance may be significantly reduced
- Don't take a drug that has expired. Its toxicity can increase drastically

DRUGS COMMONLY INVOLVED IN OVERDOSE

Alcohol, Ambien, cocaine, crack, drug cocktails, heroin, methadone, Nembutal, Seconal, Vicodan, Xanax

If the drug user faints or loses consciousness because of heroin, tranquilizers, alcohol, poppers, solvents, ecstasy, one may do the following steps:

- Place the person in the recovery position
- Check breathing. Get ready to do mouth-to-mouth resuscitation
- Call an ambulance
- Keep victim warm but not hot

If she/he become intermittently responsive, do not give her or him fluids since these can easily be aspirated and be thrown into the lungs.

THE RECOVERY POSITION

If someone has collapsed and is still breathing, do the following:

- Turn the person on to his or her front, with the head sideways on the side nearest to you
- Bend his or her upper arm and leg on the side nearest to you
- Straighten the other arm and leg

- Stay with the victim, watch his or her breathing, and tell someone to call an ambulance
- Don't place anyone in the recovery position if a head or neck injury is suspected

EMERGENCY RESUSCITATION

If the heart and the breathing have stopped, don't get emotional and **act fast**.

- Tell someone to call an ambulance
- Look inside the person's mouth and scoop out any foreign bodies or vomit
- Turn the victim on to his or her back
- Tilt the head back and lift the chin slightly to pen the airway
- Close nostrils with your thumb and finger, take a deep breath, and place your mouth over the victim's mouth
- Blow into the mouth until the chest expands
- Repeat one more time
- Feel the pulse on the side of the neck or wrist with your finger
- If none is found, start cardiac massage

CARDIAC MASSAGE

- Locate the notch at the bottom of the breastbone
- Measure two finger widths above this
- Place both hands on the middle of the breastbone and press down firmly and smoothly fifteen times, at a rate of eighty times per minute
- Keep repeating mouth-to-mouth (two breaths) and then cardiac massage (fifteen compressions) until the pulse and breathing start again or until the ambulance crew arrive and take over
- Provide rescue with any information you have about the drug or drugs the victim has taken. This can be crucial to guide the emergent medical treatment

29—ACUTE ALCOHOLIC INTOXICATION

Remember: Alcoholism can be successfully treated. Go for it!

Acute and chronic alcoholism cause a great number of medical, psychiatric, social, family, and legal complications. In this section, we'll focus on the dangers of alcohol and its capacity to cause a sudden death.

The Centers for Disease Control and Prevention's National Center for Health Statistics estimates that of people in the United States aged twelve years and older, 52% drank alcohol in the past month. Of these, 16% are binge drinkers, consuming five or more drinks on the same occasion at least once in the past month.

Emergency room physicians are busy trying to figure out how much alcohol is responsible for the patient's condition and how much other intoxicating factors are playing a role. People who drink alcohol are often taking illicit drugs (e.g., cocaine, opiates) or are intoxicated by other alcohols (e.g., methanol) and have altered mental status due to hepatic encephalopathy, head trauma, meningitis, encephalitis, sepsis, fever, stroke, gastrointestinal bleeding, respiratory failure due to aspiration or depression of respiratory drive, severe hypoglycemia (alcohol reduces the production of glucose by the liver), severe dehydration (alcohol is a natural diuretic), **and cardiac arrhythmias. Some of these can be serious and even fatal.**

DIAGNOSIS OF ALCOHOLIC INTOXICATION

Is the patient's mental status just due to alcohol intoxication or any of the above described medical conditions, alone or in various combinations?

The diagnosis of ethanol intoxication should never be made on the basis of behavior alone. Blood levels count.

One drink equals 1 oz (one shot) of 80 proof liquor, 12 oz of beer, or 4-5 oz of wine.

An ounce of 80 proof liquor in a 70 kg person raises BAC by 25 mg/dL or 5.4 mmol/L.

Alcohol consumption (drinks) Per person		Approximate BAC, mg/dL (Blood Alcohol Concentration)	Probable clinical manifestations
1-3	2-5	50-100 mg/dL	Incoordination
>10	>15	>400 mg/dL	Coma Respiratory arrest Death

Blood alcohol concentration (BAC) remains the definitive standard for assessing intoxication and is expressed in milligrams per deciliter (mg/dL).

The legal intoxication level varies by state, but in general it is 80 mg/dL. The average clearance rate in both adults and children is 18-20 mg/dL per hour. Elderly drinkers have a higher BAC than younger abusers of the same weight for any given amount of alcohol consumed.

Alcohol induces mental changes that vary from lethargic depression to violent delirium.

Agitated patients must be protected from themselves and from similarly intoxicated persons.

I was called on repeated occasions to see a thirty-six-year-old woman at the hospital ER who invariably appeared intoxicated with alcohol and physically abused by her husband, a 6'4" muscular, huge guy, a well-dressed corporate executive. Upon my arrival to the ER I always saw the husband kissing her and treating her with great deference after beating her. Her face, arms, and thorax showed extensive bruises and rib fractures. Both of her parents and her husband's parents were all alcoholics, and every time I was called, I saw six persons—the patient, her husband, her parents, and the in-laws—all intoxicated, holding hands, hugging, and consoling each other.

**

A man in his fifties suffered from severe alcoholic cardiomyopathy and had many alcoholic brothers and sisters. Why so many alcoholics in one single family? His parents died when he was an infant, and his grandmother had to take care of eleven children. They made so much noise at sleeping time that she replaced bottles of milk with bottles of beer so she could have some rest at night. All these kids became alcoholics.

**

Abe was eighty-three and was admitted to the hospital with a severe urinary tract infection. A couple of days later, he became confused and so agitated that required restrains. There was no history of alcoholism known to his wife and daughter. I wanted to rule out an alcohol withdrawal reaction, and during one of his violent reactions, I asked him: "Abe, would you like a little scotch?" He said, "You're an angel. Where is it?"

I asked his wife to bring to the hospital a bottle of whiskey. She did. He drank part of it voraciously. I couldn't have drunk tea that fast! A few minutes later, he was fully alert, cooperative, and calm. Later on, his wife discovered at home many bottles of hard liquor hidden in different places. She had never suspected that her husband was an alcoholic.

When patients are under the influence of alcohol, it is essential to rule out additional head trauma, electrolyte abnormalities, adverse reactions to illicit or prescription drugs, and other causes of mental deterioration as well as dehydration, hypoglycemia, internal bleeding, airway compromise due to suppressed protective reflexes, and lung aspiration of gastric contents.

There is no specific antidote or reversal agent for alcohol toxicity.

Treatment includes respiratory care, proper hydration, control of nausea and vomiting, correction of electrolyte deficiencies such as hypomagnesemia, glucose for hypoglycemia, thiamine supplementation.

Heavy alcohol use increases the risk of major strokes.

Heavy alcohol consumption during pregnancy is associated with an increased risk of spontaneous abortion.

Rapid ingestion of large quantities of alcohol represents a medical emergency **(alcohol poisoning)** that can quickly lead to fatal respiratory depression. Absorption mostly takes place in the small bowel, very little in the stomach, and it starts in ten minutes. Serum BAC (blood alcohol concentration) peaks between thirty and ninety minutes after ingestion. Effects are particularly severe in young, nontolerant binge drinkers. Efficient respiratory care,

Since the absorption of alcohol occurs rapidly via the intestinal mucosa, gastric lavage is of limited value although it may lower the maximum BAC if done a few minutes after alcohol ingestion.

PREVENTION OF FUTURE INTOXICATION

Every intoxicated patient should be evaluated for suicide risk. Domestic violence and homelessness need to be explored. Social service options, shelter referrals need to be available. A sober guardian is necessary. This person should be provided written instructions including warning signs of deterioration and alcohol withdrawal.

Somewhat surprisingly, about 50% of patients referred to ambulatory centers for alcoholism keep their appointments.

Alcoholics Anonymous, family counseling, detoxification units, and treatment centers are indispensable for the follow-up of patients who suffer from this addiction.

30—AMPHETAMINES, BARBITURATES, ECSTASY, MAGIC MUSHROOMS, POPPERS, VICODAN, TRANQUILIZERS, AND XANAX

AMPHETAMINES

These drugs are known in the street as Dexys Midnight Runners, phets, base, glass, uppers, whiz, billy, and sulph although the most common **popular name for amphetamine is speed.** It is a central nervous system stimulant. Chemically, it has some similarities with norepinephrine, a hormone produced by the adrenal gland in excess during stressful situations.

There are three pharmaceutical classes: levo or diamphetamine **(Benzedrine),** dextroamphetamine **(Dexedrine)** and methylamphetamine **(methedrine).** The latter is the most potent of the three.

The favorite street product is amphetamine sulphate, which is a mixture of levoamphetamine and dextroamphetamine. It's a dirty white or pinkish powder, which is snorted, rubbed on the gums, dissolved in liquid for injection or drinking. It also comes in a pill form.

Amphetamines may be "cut" with paracetamol, baby milk, talcum powder, and other substances, so the consumer really doesn't know what combination of additional poisons he or she is taking.

Amphetamines make you talk, and you become more lively, confident, and outgoing, that is, until the moment you get into trouble. The appetite may disappear. Side effects include anxiety, depression, irritability, memory and concentration impairment. It quickens the respiration and the heart rate, and users have died from overdose.

BARBITURATES

Some of the slangs for this group of drugs are these: barbs, barbies, blue bullets, blue devils, gorillas, pink ladies, red devils, sleepers.

Barbiturates have a strong sedative effect. They depress the central nervous system. Larger doses lead to speech slurring, clumsiness, and unconsciousness. Doctors prescribe them as sleeping pills. Since they were associated with too many fatalities, tranquilizers replaced them to a large extent.

Mixing barbiturates with alcohol, heroin, or tranquilizer and other substances may be fatal. Withdrawal reactions are severe (irritability, inability to sleep, nausea, convulsions). Sudden withdrawal from high doses can be lethal. Heavy users suppress the cough reflex and develop bronchitis and pneumonia as well as hypothermia.

One of the treacherous things about barbiturates is that the doses that kill are not too much higher than the doses "normally" used. Barbiturates are not only responsible for killing the user but for accidents where the user dies and takes other innocent people with him/her.

ECSTASY

The chemical abbreviation for this drug is MDMA, and the problems it causes are similar to those noted by amphetamine and cocaine users, including addiction. This drug has a stimulating effect causing euphoria and increased alertness in addition to psychedelic effects. It was first used in the 1980s and became a favorite of young people attending raves.

It is precisely in these raves where fatalities occur. Raves are large, all-night dance parties, and in the past years the use of the drug has increased in college students. The stimulant effects of ecstasy enable these deeply mistaken young fellows to dance for extended periods. And it has been observed that the drug plus the hot, crowded conditions found in raves have caused dehydration, high fever, heart and kidney failure.

Serotonin is a substance thought to play a role in regulating mood, memory, sleep, and appetite. Ecstasy damages brain serotonin cells and causes long-lasting damage to brain areas that are critical for thought and memory. These may become permanent. Ecstasy and intense dancing for hours without taking regular breaks affect the body's temperature due to overheating and dehydration. Signs include dizziness, fainting, cramps, headache, or sudden loss of energy.

A water balance is usually adequate when the water intake while on ecstasy is a pint of water or so every hour, and also relaxing and getting cooler when the person feels too hot.

MAGIC MUSHROOMS

Mushies, magics, happies, sillies, purple passion

There are two main types of magic mushrooms—the psylocybe species containing the psychoactive chemical psilocybin and psilocin while the *Amanita muscaria* variety contains ibotenic acid and muscimol as the main psychoactive ingredients.

Their effects are quite similar to those produced by LSD, but "the trip" tends to be shorter and milder (about four hours). They produce euphoria and excitement. Hallucinations can occur and can complicate preexisting mental problems.

Serious health risks and even death may result due to eating the wrong kind of mushrooms.

If you ate magic mushrooms and you don't feel well, go straight to a hospital with a sample and tell the ER practitioner how much of the mushroom you consumed.

POPPERS

This is the term for the group of chemicals known as alkyl nitrates that include amyl nitrite, butyl nitrate, and isobutyl nitrite. These are clear liquids contained in a small bottle or tube. The vapor is inhaled through the mouth or nose. **The name *poppers* derives from the noise that is produced when the nitrate container is opened.**

Amyl nitrate is stronger than butyl nitrate. Years ago, amyl nitrate was used to treat heart conditions and also during acute biliary colic attacks to relieve painful spasms.

Effects occur **fast**, immediately, and are brief (about five minutes) but intense: light-headedness, heat flush, or heightened sensual awareness may result ("head rush"). There is often a residual headache.

Poppers are popular within the club and dance culture.

THE RISKS

- Side effects of sniffing poppers include headaches, nausea, coughing, dizziness, and fainting.
- If spilled, poppers can burn the skin.
- They lower the blood pressure. Special dangers are present for those who have anemia, glaucoma, respiratory or cardiac problems.
- Low blood pressure may affect pregnant women. Nitrates cross the placenta.
- The combination of Viagra and poppers may drastically drop the blood pressure and lead to a cardiac arrest and death.
- **If swallowed, they can be fatal.**

VICODAN

This is one of the most frequently used pain medications nowadays. Related medications are lorict, Loritab, Percodan, and OxyContin and are opiod-based pain drugs.

Vicodan is usually successful in relieving pain, but it is highly addictive, and withdrawal symptoms can be severe.

Symptoms of Vicodan overdose include bluish tinge in skin; blood disorders; cold and clammy skin; heavy perspiration; heart, kidney, and liver problems; vomiting; and respiratory difficulties. A severe overdose of Vicodan can be fatal.

TRANQUILIZERS

Slang terms: benzos, eggs, jellies, norries

Some products names include Valium, Ativan, Librium, Mogadon. Chemical names include diazepam, lorazepam, nitrazepam, chlordiazepoxide, flunitrazepam, temazepam.

These drugs are prescribed for anxiety, stress, tension problems, and sleeping disorders. Some people mix them with heroin and alcohol. They come in capsules, tablets, or in injectable form. Higher than indicated doses cause drowsiness, and the effects last from 3 to 6 hours. Withdrawal may cause insomnia and convulsions.

If combined with other drugs, specially alcohol, fatal overdose can occur.

XANAX

It is used to treat disorders related to anxiety and stress. People take it to suppress unwanted feelings and thoughts. Xanax addiction progresses quickly. When abused, it is taken orally, chewed, crushed, then snorted like cocaine, or crushed then dissolved in water and injected like heroin.

Xanax has a depressant effect and impairs alertness like alcohol or sedative barbiturates do.

This drug can be dangerous when overdose happens. The consumer looks for the "high" feeling and doesn't realize that the difference between the doses necessary to feel that way and the doses that produces death is small.

An overdose of Xanax taken alone or in combination with alcohol can be fatal.

31—COCAINE

An old Indian goddess becomes a vulgar street villain.

Cocaine, Mama Coca, was, in fact, considered by South American Indians as a sacred goddess, a benevolent deity who blessed humans with her powers. Cocaine leaves were used for at least 5,000 years. In pre-Columbian times, these were reserved for Inca royalty. The natives finally used it for mystical, religious, social, nutritional, and medical purposes.

This plant, that in its native habitat is resistant to drought and disease, needs no irrigation and can be harvested several times a year, has stimulating properties, enhances endurance, wards off fatigue and hunger, and produces a sense of well-being. It was initially banished by the Spanish conquistadores. But the Incas could barely work the fields or gold mines without it, so addicted they were to it. So the Catholic Church decided to cultivate it. Coca leaves were distributed three to four times a day during brief rest breaks. The conquistadores themselves finally came to like it too and imported it to Europe. The "elixir of life" had finally arrived!

In 1814, an editorial in *Gentleman's Magazine* urged researchers to begin experimentation so that coca could be used as "a substitute for food, so that people could live a month, now and then, without eating."

Cocaine was first synthesized around 1860 from the leaves of the coca plant (*Erythroxylon*). At that time, it was thought to be a wonder drug capable of curing many illnesses. Cocaine was sold over the counter until 1916. One could buy it at stores. Harrods was one of them. Anyone could buy a cocaine chocolate tablet. The huge laboratory Parke-Davis announced that cocaine "could make the coward brave, the silent eloquent, and render the sufferer insensitive to pain." Sigmund Freud, the pioneer of psychoanalysis, began to experiment with cocaine in the early 1880s. He liked it so much that he wrote several scientific articles about it. In fact, he was paid by giant pharmaceutical corporations for his endorsement of cocaine.

John Pemberton was a druggist from Atlanta, Georgia, who badly wanted to create a national drink, and spent years of hard work trying to come up with a formula using coca leaves. When he got it right, he named it Coca-Cola, but he was in his fifties and had a terminal illness. He sold it for little money, and his wife died a pauper a few years later. Those who bought the formula from him did very well indeed.

The Coca-Cola sold today still contains an extract of coca leaves, but these are used only for flavoring since the drug has been removed. In the nineteenth century, popular drinks with coca leaf extracts were launched into the market, and celebrities not only drank them but endorsed them. There was public praise for them from Queen Victoria, Thomas Edison, the pope, and other celebrities.

Since 1980s, cocaine has become a significant export earner for some poor South American countries, mostly Peru and Bolivia. In the year 2000, South America exported 1,000 tons of refined cocaine.

Today, cocaine is a Schedule II drug. This means that it has high potential for abuse but can be used by a doctor for legitimate medical situations, such as a local anesthetic for some eye, ear, and throat surgeries.

There are two chemical forms of cocaine: cocaine hydrochloride, or powder form of cocaine, dissolves in water and can be taken intravenously (by vein) or intranasally (through the nose). The freebase cocaine can be smoked.

Cocaine is generally known in the street as coke, C, flake, blow, and snow.

In the United States, 5 million people report using cocaine annually on a regular basis, and in 2003 alone, 34.9 million Americans (including those as young as twelve years of age) reported using cocaine at least once.

Cocaine is the most frequently abused drug in patients presenting to emergency departments and is the most frequent cause of drug-related deaths reported by medical examiners. Although cocaine can be detected in blood or urine for only a few hours, its metabolites or degradation products can be detected for 24-36 hours after ingestion. Biochemical analysis of hair is a very sensitive marker of cocaine use in the preceding months. Cocaine is highly addictive.

HOW COCAINE MAY CAUSE CARDIOVASCULAR DAMAGE AND DEATH

Cocaine increases the heart rate, blood pressure, and the contractility of the heart. This may create an imbalance between the amount of blood that is supplied to the heart and what the heart muscle needs. When the needs are higher than the demands, a **myocardial infarction** may develop.

* **Procoagulation effect**. Cocaine increases platelet adhesiveness, and this increases the tendency to clot formation inside the arteries and the veins. The latter may occur in the lower extremities but **occasionally the patient presents with a swollen arm due to subclavian vein thrombosis. Any person who presents with this abnormality should be immediately suspected as being a cocaine user**
* **Vasospasm** occurs, and this vasoconstriction deprives the heart muscle of adequate blood supply and may lead to **acute myocardial infarction**

* **Accelerated atherosclerosis.** Coronary artery disease is typically found in 35% to 55% of patients undergoing coronary angiography for cocaine-associated chest pain
* **Deterioration of left ventricular dysfunction**: Cocaine may cause acute or chronic weakness of the heart muscle leading to congestive heart failure
* **Serious arrhythmias** are seen in some patients. Some rhythms are chaotic and lead to **ventricular fibrillation**
* **Endocarditis.** This results from the intravenous use of cocaine. The mitral and aortic valves are most frequently affected
* **Aortic dissection.** This diagnosis should be entertained in any patient with cocaine-associated chest pain. Cocaine-induced catecholamine surge leads to elevated shear-stress forces. This increases the proclivity for tears and aortic dissection. Dissection of coronary arteries has also been documented

The patient's chest pains may temporarily improve with nitroglycerin and calcium blockers, but these patients need to be observed carefully and treated in a hospital environment. Psychological support and drug addiction management is essential. Many cocaine users are also addicted to other drugs, and **the combination of cocaine and alcohol addiction is particularly dangerous.**

I was once asked to take care of Walter, an eighteen-year-old boy, who was in critical condition at the ER of a major hospital. The picture looked gloomy from the start. He was in coma, the left side of his body was paralyzed, he had shallow respirations and very low blood pressure. He died from cocaine and alcohol intoxication in forty-eight hours. His "friends" gave him a farewell party. Next day he was supposed to fly to California to start his college studies. He consumed cocaine, alcohol, and other unidentified drugs. I called his parents, his three brothers and two sisters, let them see the cadaver, and advised the teenagers to take a hard look at the beautiful boy now in his way to cremation, hoping that they would avoid a similar tragedy by not taking drugs of any kind, alcohol, and also to learn how to select mentally and emotionally healthy friends and acquaintances.

A few days later, I received in the mail a thank-you card with Walter's photo embracing his dog, and this inscription: "From Walter and his family, during happier times!"

This was one of saddest cases I had to deal with in my professional life.

32—EPHEDRA

Ephedra is a substance obtained from a plant (*Ephedra sinica*) that has been used in China for thousands of years for the treatment of asthma and hay fever. Mormons and American Indians drank a tea brewed from an ephedra called Mormon tea.

Ephedra was found to cause serious side effects, death included. The FDA banned the sale of ephedra-containing supplements on April 12, 2004. This decision was legally appealed, but the ban on ephedra was upheld. Since June 2007, the sale of ephedra-containing supplements has been illegal.

Ephedra has been used to reduce appetite in combination with caffeine and aspirin and also by athletes although it doesn't affect physical performance. Side effects of ephedra may include skin rashes, nervousness, insomnia, excessive perspiration, high fever, seizures, palpitations, a heart attack, stroke, and death.

Ephedra-related adverse reactions were reviewed in a 2000 issue of the *New England Journal of Medicine* where this drug was noted to be related to a number of cases of death and disability, many of which occurred in young adults who used ephedra in the labeled dosages.

33—HEROIN

A distressingly frequent and awful miscalculation.

Heroin is an illegal, highly addictive drug. It is the most rapidly acting and the most abused of the opiates. This drug is characteristically sold as a white or brown powder or as the black sticky substance known on the street as black tar heroin. Street names include smack, H, skag, and junk. Heroin is extracted from morphine, which in turn comes from the seedpod of the Asian poppy plant.

Most street heroin is "cut" with other substances such as sugar, starch, quinine, powder milk, strychnine, or other dangerous poisons. Users and abusers don't have the vaguest idea about the strength or contaminants contained in this product, and **every time they consume it, they are at risk of death.** Sharing needles is a common occurrence in heroin addicts, and the risk of HIV, hepatitis, and other infections is an ever-present possibility.

Heroin can be injected, sniffed/snorted, or smoked. Snorters sometimes shift to needle injecting because of increased tolerance, nasal soreness, or unreliable purity. A typical heroin abuser may inject up to four times a day. Intravenous injection provides the greatest intensity and most rapid of euphoria (7-8 seconds) while intramuscular injection produces a slower onset of euphoria (5-8 minutes). When this drug is snored or sniffed, the peak effects are felt within 10-15 minutes. Any form of heroin administration is highly addictive.

In some sectors of society, heroin is available in high purity and inexpensive form. This has attracted younger users across the United States. After the initial euphoric effects, abusers feel drowsy for several hours, and mental function is altered. Respiration is badly affected, and cardiac function becomes impaired. Sometimes death follows.

In pregnancy, heroin can cause miscarriage and premature delivery. Children born to addicted mothers are at greater risk of SIDS (sudden infant death syndrome). Drug treatment with methadone is advised. Infants born to mothers taking prescribed methadone may show signs of physical dependence but can be treated safely in the nursery.

Acute heroin overdose is a common cause of preventable death. In urban and suburban localities in the United States, heroin overdose is a daily experience. The central nervous system is rapidly affected. The user has an abnormal mental status, respiration is depressed, and pupils are small (miotic). Most overdoses occur at home, in the company of others, and usually there are other drugs involved as well. Heroin-related deaths are strongly associated with the concomitant use of alcohol. In fact, **it takes lower doses of heroin to kill a person who is highly intoxicated with alcohol.**

In persons who regularly inject heroin, the average annual mortality rate is 2%. Half of this rate is attributable to overdose. This rate is 6-20 times the mortality rate expected in non-drug-user peers.

Heroin is seven times more toxic than morphine when given intravenously. The route of administration influences the deadly outcome. **Most fatal heroin overdoses occur when the drug is given intravenously although a small number of heroin-related deaths have been associated with intranasal administration.**

Most deaths occur in users who are in their late twenties to early thirties, have used heroin for 5-10 years, and are highly dependent on the drug, and take place 1-3 hours after injection. **Instant death does not appear to be the rule. This observation is important because it gives the victim the opportunity to go or be taken to a hospital emergency room for treatment with naloxone.** Most patients have inadequate respiration and should receive bag-valve-mask ventilation followed by naloxone within 5-20 minutes of administration. Failure of adequate response to respiratory impairment may require the use of endotracheal intubation. One to three percent of patients with heroin overdose develop pulmonary edema, which is not related to heart failure.

In patients with heroin overdose, naloxone is associated with a 1.6% rate of serious complications, including seizures and arrhythmias. **Many abusers fail to call an ambulance because of fear of police involvement.**

And now, the good news is this: heroin addicts can change the behaviors that put them at risk of contracting HIV and other infections. They can also be successfully treated to eliminate the drug use.

34—METHADONE

Slangs: Juice, green, meth, phy

Methadone is a synthetic drug with pain-killing properties. It works like heroin though it is less addictive. This is the reason for using methadone as a substitute to help the withdrawal symptoms of those addicted to heroin. It is a green liquid preparation although it also available in tablet or injection.

This drug is only available on prescription. The effects are similar to those of heroin, Drowsiness can occur when methadone is taken in higher than recommended doses, and the effects last up to twenty-four hours, which is longer than heroin. Those who are treated for heroin addiction do not have the need to take methadone as often as they need to take heroin. **Methadone is in itself a highly addictive drug. Although it may help to correct the heroin addiction, it may create its own dependency problems.** Unsupervised withdrawal may lead to insomnia, vomiting, cold and hot sweats, and cramps. **Methadone is a powerful and dangerous drug. High doses may lead to coma and death.**

35—VIAGRA, LEVITRA, AND CIALIS

These drugs have an extraordinary safety record, and although they may have certain side effects, they are usually well tolerated. The big mistake would be to take any of these drugs with nitroglycerin or nitrate derivatives. Nitroglycerin is used in tablets, sprays, ointments, pastes, patches, and it is also used intravenously. Nitrate derivatives can also be found in other medicines (e.g., isosorbide dinitrate or isosorbide mononitrate). Some recreational drugs called poppers also contain nitrates, such as amyl nitrate and butyl nitrite.

Do not use Viagra, Levitra, or Cialis if you are using these drugs. A precipitous fall in the blood pressure might occur, and it could be severe enough to cause a cardiac arrest. That is not the medication's fault, but the mistake of combining it with the wrong drug.

Patients who have low blood pressure due to other reasons, e.g., dehydration, blood pressure medications that dropped the blood pressure to undesirable low levels, the so-called orthostatic hypotension syndrome where the blood pressure drop is so severe that leads to fainting, **should also avoid Viagra, Levitra, or Cialis. Always seek medical counseling before using these drugs. Never take them without a health care practitioner authorization, and do not allow any of your "friends" to give you any of these pills for you to try and see how it works.**

36—PHENOTHIAZINES

Some of the following are phenothiazine derivatives: Stelazine, Compazine, Phenergan, Thorazine, promazine, Mellaril, Prolixin, Triavil, Trilafon.

Phenothiazine is a chemical frequently used in the manufacture of antipsychotic drugs. It was introduced as an insecticide in 1935, and it is used in the manufacture of rubber derivatives in the chemical industry, and it is used as an antiparasitic agent in livestock. Phenothiazines is a term used to describe the largest of the five main classes of neuroleptic antipsychotic drugs. These medications often have antiemetic properties (relieve nausea) although they are capable of causing rigidity of the extremities and tremors.

Neuroleptic is a term that refers to the effects of antipsychotic drugs on a patient, especially in his/her behavior. Neuroleptic drugs produce apathy. Psychotic patients reduce their confusion and agitation.

Rarely neuroleptic drugs produce the so-called neuroleptic malignant syndrome (NMS) which is potentially fatal. Characteristically, this syndrome presents with fever, muscular rigidity, and delirium.

37—PROARRHYTHMIC EFFECTS OF SOME NONCARDIAC DRUGS

A number of noncardiac drugs used to treat many different medical conditions are capable of causing life-threatening arrhythmias. One of them is the so-called "torsade de pointes": This is a rhythm disturbance where the ventricle generates an intrusive and highly abnormal electrical phenomenon with a burst of very fast and very irregular beats, which have the potential to degenerate into another arrhythmia, which is even worse, namely, ventricular fibrillation, a chaotic cardiac rhythm that ends in death unless it is quickly reversed.

It is important to remember that many useful medications, including those capable of inducing "torsade de pointes", can be medically used with benefit to the patient. An infrequent side effect, even although it may be a very important one such as the arrhythmia described here, should not deter the doctor and the patient from using a drug that has been selected after a careful evaluation and good medical judgment. The physician makes a choice of a medication after concluding that the benefits of using one particular drug exceed its potential to cause an infrequent but serious side effect.

These are some of the medications that have been observed to be associated with torsade de pointes: terfenadine, astemizole, cisapride, macrolides, fluroquinolones, antimalarials, antifungals, tricyclic antidepressants, antipsychotics.

38—PROARRHYTHMIC EFFECTS OF CARDIAC DRUGS

The use of cardiac drugs has revolutionized the treatment of heart disease. Medications used to treat heart failure or arrhythmias are extraordinarily useful, and generally, they are used without significant side effects. These are controlled by reducing the doses of the drug or replacing it with another one.

Paradoxically, the very same medications that suppress certain arrhythmias may at times cause them. Does it sound crazy? Yes, it does, but that's the way it is!

If you have a cardiac disorder and expect any cardiac medication to assure you it would never cause an important or even dangerous side effect, you are on the wrong side of the equation. All cardiac drugs (and many non-cardiac drugs) have a potential for serious side effects. When you accept to take a cardiac medication, you do it because the potential advantages and benefits override its potential dangers. In other words, the risks from not taking the medication are greater than the risks from taking it.

Digitalis, procainamide, quinidine, fleicanide, beta-blockers, amiodarone, calcium antagonists, flecainamide, propafenone, and others may rarely be fatal. Cardiologists correctly use these drugs all the time, and the vast majority of patients respond well to them and avoid suffering, disability, or a premature death.

39—NASAL VASOCONSTRICTORS (DROPS FOR A RUNNING NOSE)

Millions of people use nose drops for rhinitis (inflammation of the nasal mucosa) for bad colds, allergies, or chronic rhinitis. These substances are absorbed from the nasal mucosa into the bloodstream. They act locally by constricting the small blood vessels. By doing so, secretions are reduced.

The trouble with this vasoconstrictive effect is that it does not only occur in the nasal mucosa but throughout the body and may affect the cerebral or cardiac circulation and cause a great deal of trouble.

I once treated a forty-two-year-old patient who nearly lost his life from the vascular spasms induced by nose drops containing pseudoephedrine, which he grossly abused trying to suppress his profuse nasal secretions. In the process, he almost suppressed himself.

He was brought by an ambulance to the hospital emergency room because of severe chest pains. Minutes after his arrival, the left side of his body paralyzed, and the electrocardiogram showed a massive acute myocardial infarction. His paralysis disappeared in a couple of hours. His coronary angiogram showed "normal" coronary arteries. The mechanism thought to be the likely cause of his temporary stroke was a spasm of the carotid-cerebral circulation. The heart attack was the result of an intense coronary artery spasm. He survived. He told me that he had been dripping into his nostrils "gallons a day" of nose drops containing pseudoephedrine.

This medication, in normal doses, administered in pill or nose drops form may cause coronary artery constriction in an occasional patient. Those who suffer from coronary atherosclerosis and narrowing of the coronary arteries should avoid them altogether.

PART 5

HEART DISEASE

A sudden death that could have been prevented is, to say the least, twice as tragic.

40—SUDDEN CARDIAC DEATH (SCD), CARDIAC ARREST, AND CARDIOPULMONARY RESUSCITATION (CPR), VENTRICULAR TACHYCARDIA (VT), VENTRICULAR FIBRILLATION (VF), AND CARDIAC STANDSTILL

Sudden cardiac death (SCD) is an unexpected natural death due to a cardiac cause that occurs in the presence of heart disease, unrecognized heart disease, or absence of preexisting heart disease. The victim may have preceding symptoms, such as shortness of breath, chest pains, palpitations, or no symptoms whatsoever. The person collapses, and death follows. The time from the onset of the event and death is one hour or less although some authorities extend this period to less than two hours. SCD is preceded by a cardiac arrest.

Cardiac arrest is the sudden cessation of effective cardiac contractions. The most common mechanism for SCD is an arrhythmia, generally **ventricular tachycardia (VT),** a fast rhythm that originates in the ventricle instead of the normal place, which is the sinus node located at the right atrium, or **ventricular fibrillation (VF),** which is a chaotic rhythm, characterized by weak, feeble, totally ineffective cardiac muscle contractions: the left ventricle is unable to pump blood into the general circulation. Vital organs do not receive the necessary blood supply for their functioning. The brain is one of them. This is what produces unconsciousness.

Ventricular fibrillation is the first recorded rhythm in approximately 75% of patients who have a cardiac arrest. Twenty to thirty percent of patients from all documented sudden death events have very slow heart rhythms (severe bradycardia). Sometimes, there's no rhythm at all: the ECG shows a straight line (no electrical cardiac activity). This is called **asystole or cardiac standstill.**

In the United States alone, there are more than 400,000 sudden cardiac deaths yearly. **Eighty percent of SCDs occur in the home environment.** The average age of SCD victims is around sixty-five years. As age advances, so do the accompanying cardiac arrests. SCD has a much higher incidence in men than in women. In between 45 and 64 years of age, male to female ratio is 7:1 but drops to 2:1 in persons 65-74 years.

SCD accounts for 20% of all sudden deaths in patients younger than twenty years of age. The incidence of SCD is higher in Afro Americans than in whites. Asians are the least likely candidates to suffer this condition.

Almost as many as 50% of patients who have a SCD have been seen by a physician within four weeks before death, and most of their complaints had no connection with the heart.

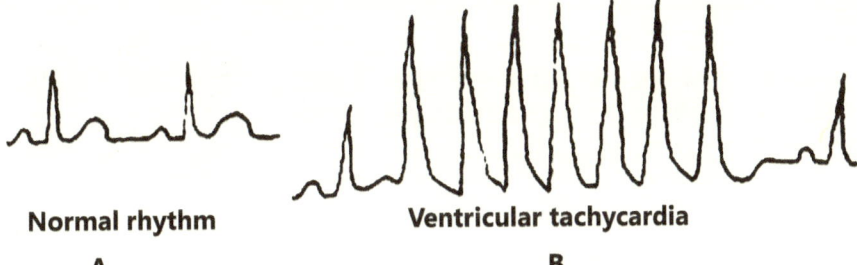

Normal rhythm

A

Ventricular tachycardia

B

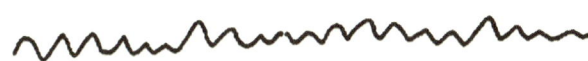

Special kind of ventricular tachycardia
Torsade de pointes

C

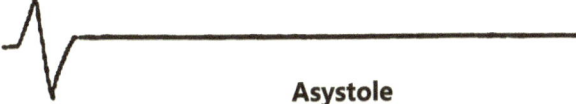

Ventricular fibrillation

D

Asystole

E

Figure 7

CORONARY ARTERY DISEASE

Most cases of SCD are due to atherosclerosis of the coronary arteries (plaques that contain lipids [fats] and calcium that are distributed throughout the arterial system, in preferential locations, the coronary arteries being one of them).

SCD is frequently the first expression of coronary artery disease and is responsible for approximately 50% of all deaths from coronary arteriosclerosis. The usual case is to find at least two major coronary arteries with severe blockages (75-85% of the arterial lumen).

A high incidence of SCD occurs in those with weakened heart muscles and ejection fraction less than 30-35%, whether this poorly functioning heart muscle resulted from an acute myocardial infarction or something else.

SCD also takes place in the presence of completely normal coronary arteries due to other cardiac disturbances.

Are coronary atherosclerotic plaques significant only when they obstruct the artery significantly, e.g., 75% or more?

The answer is *no*! And this is the explanation: A coronary artery may have a mild lesion, such as a narrowing of 20% and lead to a SCD. Why? Because the plaque is soft and vulnerable, it is susceptible to a crack or fissure, and when that happens, a clot is formed (thrombus) and may block the lumen (place where the blood circulates) of the artery completely. The result is a potentially deadly arrhythmia, which is associated—or not—with an acute myocardial infarction.

Sometimes a lethal arrhythmia ends a person's life so quickly that the heart doesn't have enough time to develop a myocardial infarction.

THE IMPORTANCE OF YOUR LIFESTYLE

I've discussed cardiovascular risk factors in a separate section of this book. Please see section 125.

Prevention of a sudden cardiac death includes radical modification of correctable cardiovascular risk factors, such as improper nutrition, inadequate physical activities, avoidance of smoking or excessive alcohol consumption, stress reduction, normalizing body weight, keeping the blood pressure and blood lipids levels where they should be, correcting elevated levels of homocysteine.

A person's ignorance on basic health issues is not usually listed in cardiology treaties as a major cardiovascular risk factor. I personally believe that **neglect and ignorance are the most important ones.** Many patients have no knowledge or vague, superficial notions about atherosclerosis, where it starts and where it ends. Some have that knowledge, but fail to apply it.

Most people know their social security number, but when you ask them about their cholesterol blood levels, HDL, LDL, or triglycerides levels, they ignore them. Everybody should know these numbers.

NON-ATHEROSCLEROTIC DISEASE OF THE CORONARY ARTERIES

There are diseases of the coronary arteries that are not atherosclerotic and are capable of causing a SCD. I'll briefly describe them in the next pages.

- Coronary artery embolization
- Coronary artery blockage due to hematological disorder
- Coronary artery spasm (e.g., cocaine use)
- Coronary obstruction due to thickening of the arterial wall (e.g., radiation therapy)
- Inborn errors of metabolism (e.g., mucopolysaccharidoses)
- Congenital coronary artery anomalies (anomalous origin of a coronary artery, coronary fistula
- Coronary artery dissection
- Congenital and acquired coronary aneurysm
- Infectious coronary arteritis: tuberculosis, typhoid, syphilis viruses
- Noninfectious coronary arteritis: Kawasaki disease, Takayasu arteritis, giant cell arteritis (temporal arteritis), SLE (systemic lupus erythematosus), rheumatoid arthritis, ankylosing spondilitis, thromboangiitis obliterans, polyarteritis nodosa
- Allergic vasculitis
- Coronary artery trauma
- Myocardial oxygen demand-supply imbalance

Other heart diseases that increase the risk of SCD will be discussed below.

CARDIOPULMONARY RESUSCITATION (CPR)

Of the 400,000 people who have SCD in the United States every year, 40% of them are unwitnessed. This is important because the survival of a person who suffered a cardiac arrest depends on the presence of competent individuals who can immediately call for help (911), proceed with CPR and basic life support, defibrillate the patient as soon as possible, and have the patient taken to the nearest hospital for advanced cardiac support.

Cardiac arrests are living (or dying) tragedies. For decades, great efforts were invested in trying to resuscitate these patients and keeping them alive. Despite the better understanding we have these days to proceed with cardiopulmonary resuscitation (CPR), the final results are deceptive.

Out-of-hospital cardiac arrests that are not treated with early defibrillation do very poorly. In New York, Los Angeles, and Chicago the survival from out-of-hospital cardiac arrests is about 1%.

THE MOUTH-TO-MOUTH CPR STORY

For many decades, I was involved in CPR efforts on multiple occasions. Making rounds in hospitals meant the moral-professional obligation to respond to a call from the hospital operator through a loud speaker: "Yellow Code, Yellow Code, Yellow Code, third floor . . ." I'd run to reach a patient I had never met with a cardiac arrest, either lying in bed or on the floor. Cardiac massage, assisted ventilation, and quite a few years ago, intracardiac injections of adrenaline were part of the reviving effort.

The mouth-to-mouth breathing was unpleasant, to put it mildly. There was a direct contact between my mouth and the victim's mouth. Some patients had vomited, others had the smell of spaghetti sauce or cucumbers, and I dutifully did the best I could to overcome my distaste for the mouth-to-mouth contact and went ahead with the procedure anyway.

Recently, major changes in CPR technique were made, and it is now realized that the ventilation contribution during CPR, namely,

breathing into the patient's mouth, alternating with cardiac compression, is not only unnecessary, but on many occasions, it may be harmful.

Ventilations or "rescue breathing" is considered important in cardiac arrest **when a respiratory problem is the cause of it. So it is extremely important to use ventilation efforts in those whose cardiac arrest resulted from asphyxia.**

There's an important difference between a "primary" cardiac arrest, namely, an arrest caused by a cardiac cause than a cardiac arrest that resulted from "hypoxia," namely, low concentration of oxygen in the blood due to an untreated respiratory arrest. In this latter situation, the arterial blood gases show gross abnormalities and a low arterial blood oxygen concentration. These severe changes in oxygen concentration are not seen in the primary cardiac arrest situation.

So when the patient's respiratory deficiency is due to a piece of food lodged into the trachea, the Heimlich maneuver is mandatory, and assisted ventilation is critical in patients with respiratory depression due to drug overdose or other causes.

New guidelines for CPR have been offered by the American Heart Association (AHA), and I strongly urge you to contact the AHA and expand your knowledge on CPR by reading their excellent explanations, methods, and recommendations.

The recommended hand position for chest compressions is also simplified and is "the center of the chest at the nipple line."

The first phase of VF, also called the **electrical phase,** lasts for about 4-5 minutes, and the most important intervention is **rapid defibrillation.** Although the heart is fibrillating, the heart muscle (myocardium) has not yet exhausted its energy stores or suffered serious cellular damage. So the heart has good chances to respond to the defibrillator shock and generate a viable cardiac rhythm. **This is one of the reasons why AEDs (automated electrical defibrillators) have been used successfully in certain settings, such as casinos, airports, airplanes, and communities where prompt defibrillation is possible.**

The second phase of the cardiac arrest is called the **circulatory phase.** It occurs when ventricular fibrillation (VF) lasts from about 5 to 15 minutes.

Here, some of the myocardial energy stores becomes somewhat depleted, and there is accumulation of toxic metabolic products. **Defibrillation during this stage usually *does not* restore a useful rhythm** (useful rhythm is one that allows the heart to contract and eject blood into the circulation).

So it is critical to generate adequate coronary circulation with chest compressions prior to and immediately after the defibrillation attempt. Chest compressions also increase the size of the fibrillation waves, and this makes them more susceptible to respond to defibrillating electric shocks.

The third phase of the VF evolution during cardiac arrest is the **metabolic phase** of VF. After fifteen minutes, if VF persists, conversion attempts are definitely and uniformly poor. **Therefore, to treat a cardiac arrest, rapid diagnosis and treatment is essential. Cardiac arrest that is not reversed results in permanent brain damage.**

Early defibrillation is critical. Each minute that defibrillation is delayed reduces the chances of the affected person by about 10%.

Since most cardiac arrests occur in the home environment, having a defibrillator at home may be a life or death issue.

Transportation to a hospital is important, but once the cardiac arrest is diagnosed, the major emphasis should be focused in providing CPR and calling 911. If at all possible, rescue should stabilize the patient before transporting him/her to the emergency department.

Basic CPR skills can be acquired with little education and training. Of course, there are varying degrees of CPR training, and the more a rescuer knows about the subject, the greater the chances for a successful resuscitation.

Any person who is capable of learning basic CPR should be taught how to perform it.

The first thing that is needed to deal with a cardiac arrest is to make sure the patient is having a cardiac arrest:

Years ago, I arrived at the university hospital for teaching rounds with students, interns, and residents. I saw a couple of medical students and an intern doing CPR in a patient who allegedly was having ventricular fibrillation. One of them tried to do chest compressions, and the patient screamed with pain and said, "Wait a minute. Stop it! What are you doing to me?" The student obsessively continued his attempts to squeeze the patient's thorax. Trying to prevent a disruption of the team in charge of the resuscitation effort, I opted for a watchful attitude. The ECG monitor, indeed, showed what clearly appeared to be ventricular fibrillation. Seconds later, I realized that there was a physical impossibility in the patient and his deadly arrhythmia: No one having VF is responsive. A person with VF is out, flat, unconscious.

I told the student and intern: "Hold it! Stop what you're doing. This man does not have ventricular fibrillation."
"The monitor shows it!" the student said.
"That's true! However, no person who is having ventricular fibrillation is able to fight the rescuers and scream like that. Stop what you're doing!"

They did! Right there, I saw that the patient was having a tremor of his right hand. That produced an artifact in the ECG monitor screen that looked exactly like ventricular fibrillation. But of course, it was not!! The patient was more alive than you and me!

Cardiac arrest should be suspected every time a person collapses. If there's no suspicion of trauma, the unresponsive victim should be placed in supine position on a firm surface.

If there's an available ECG equipment that can identify whether the patient has standstill, ventricular tachycardia (VT), or ventricular fibrillation (VF), an ECG strip can be taken. **Nevertheless, CPR should not be delayed in favor of an electrocardiographic proof of rhythm documentation. Most cases of cardiac arrest show VF, and survival critically depends upon the duration of VF. This lethal rhythm must be eliminated fast!**

Chest Compression

In the last several years, important changes were made in the guidelines for advanced cardiac life support.

Chest compression prior to defibrillation results in improved survival during the circulatory phase of ventricular fibrillation. This is when

VF has been present for 4-5 minutes, and the rescue team arrives at the scene.

Initiation of bystander CPR and early intervention more than doubles the odds of survival following cardiac arrest.

Early defibrillation by nonmedical personnel has been advocated. Information by the general public as well the widespread availability of automated external defibrillators (AEDs) is at the crux of the problem.

It is considered that the application of a defibrillator discharge of 200 J is safe and effective for defibrillation. At times, higher discharges may be required.

Several chest positions of the electrodes to deliver the electrical discharge proved to be effective, and some people may respond better to one variant or another. The position of the electrodes most frequently used is one for the area of the tip of the heart and the other over the high right parasternal region (just to the right of the sternal bone).

Electrodes should not be placed directly over the site of implanted pacemaker or defibrillator generator.

It's been recommended by the Association for the Advancement of Medical Instrumentation a total area for both electrodes of at least 150 cm^2.

Gels or pastes should not be smeared across the chest between paddle electrodes because the electrical current may be deflected away from the heart.

A single defibrillator shock (rather than the three shocks previously recommended) is to be followed immediately by two minutes of chest compressions prior to rhythm checks. Rescuers should not check the rhythm or a pulse immediately after shock delivery—they should immediately resume CPR, beginning with chest compressions and should check the rhythm after two minutes of CPR.

The recommendation of delivering a single shock instead of the previously recommended three shocks is based on the following:

•   New defibrillators have a high success rate of conversion of VF.

- If the first shock fails, chest compressions may improve oxygen delivery to the myocardium, resulting in more likely conversion of VF with a subsequent shock.

CHEST COMPRESSION AND SURVIVAL RATES

Chest compression must be done properly to be effective. **Mouth-to-mouth ventilation remains essential for victims of respiratory arrest, but it actually decreases the likelihood of a "rescue" in those with a primary cardiac arrest.**

Mouth-to-mouth positive ventilations for primary cardiac arrest are counterproductive for these reasons:

- Some bystanders are reluctant to perform this maneuver, and therefore, truly useful resuscitation efforts are delayed or not initiated
- Both observational and experimental studies have reported improved survival with cardiac arrests who receive chest compression only as compared with those who received no chest compression until the rescue team arrived at the scene
- When a single bystander does both the compression and mouth-to-mouth ventilatory effort, the interruptions made to ventilate the patient restrict and diminish the effectiveness of chest compressions
- Mouth-to-mouth ventilation or other positive-pressure ventilation method increases the intrathoracic venous pressures. This reduces the return of venous blood to the thorax. A reduction of venous blood reaching the chest means that the left ventricle will also receive a deficient amount of blood. This compromises the coronary and cerebral blood flows. This phenomenon is particularly aggravated when a forceful ventilation is given while the chest is being compressed
- Mouth-to-mouth ventilation is not necessary in many victims of cardiac arrest because the patient's gasping provides acceptable degree of ventilation
- There is experimental evidence supporting the fact that induced cardiac arrest survival correlates best with adequate coronary and cerebral blood flow when chest compressions were used during resuscitation
- In swine studies, it has been shown that cardiac arrest survival only with chest compressions is dramatically better than with previously

guidelines recommendations of ventilations plus chest compressions when the compressions were interrupted for sixteen seconds to provide the two mouth-to-mouth breaths between each set of fifteen chest compressions

- It is estimated that the survival was twice as great in those who received bystander chest compression alone than in those who received chest compression plus mouth-to-mouth ventilation

Conclusion: Reserve CPR with chest compression plus ventilatory assistance for respiratory arrest and chest compressions only for cardiac arrest.

During a cardiac arrest, chest compressions generate improved blood flow to the brain and the heart, both of which are so badly needed. **These chest compressions must be provided without interruption until the return of spontaneous circulation or the termination of the resuscitation effort.**

ANATOMY OF THE RESUSCITATION EFFORT

Cardiac resuscitation has three components:

- The lay component for the public
- The call for rescue
- The postresuscitation component

Bystanders are instructed to call 911 to activate the emergency system as fast as possible, begin continuous chest compressions, and then, use an AED (automated electrical defibrillator), if available.

Bystanders are taught to place the heel of one hand in the center of the patient's chest, with the heel of the other on top of the first, lock the elbows so the arms are straight and fall to the weight of their upper body compressing the patient's chest.

The recommended compression rate is 100 per minute (60 compressions per minute are not adequate. The minimum should be 80 per minute. Lifting of the hands completely off the chest after each compression to allow full chest recoil is mandatory. The maneuver causes fatigue, so if more than one rescuer is present they should alternate doing chest compressions after each 100-200 compressions.

Full chest recoil during the release phase of each chest compression is essential. During the decompression (the release phase of the chest compression), a negative pressure is generated within the chest. This draws venous blood back into the right cardiac chambers and also draws air into the airways. Poor technique about this full chest recoil and decompression is critical. Not done properly, the blood flow to the brain and the coronary arteries will be severely compromised.

Special rescuers who are equipped with AEDs are to defibrillate immediately **only** if they personally witness the collapse or if good continuous chest compressions are being provided by a bystander when they arrive.

If only one rescuer is present, the defibrillator pads are quickly attached before chest compressions are started. If two rescuers are present, one begins chest compressions while the other attaches the defibrillator pads.

If a rhythm is considered potentially correctable by an electric shock applied by a defibrillator in VT (ventricular tachycardia) or VF (ventricular fibrillation), a single defibrillation current is delivered immediately. This is followed by 200 chest compressions after which rhythm and pulse analysis are carried out. These 200 compressions are done because the coronary arteries will be delivered more blood. and any attempt to defibrillate the patient again will enhance the chances of producing an effective rhythm.

Three sequential electric shocks that were recommended until recently are no longer recommended.

After the compressions were provided, the rescue team may implement other interventions, such as intravenous injections of epinephrine, amiodarone IV bolus for recurrent VT, high flow oxygen, oral-pharyngeal airway and positive pressure ventilation.

I recommend you to expand your knowledge on this subject by visiting the Web sites of the American Heart Association and the American Red Cross or contacting these organizations. They provide excellent guidelines.

CAUSES OF SUDDEN OR RAPID CARDIAC DEATH

CORONARY ARTERY BLOCKAGES DUE TO ATHEROSCLEROSIS AND OTHER NON-ATHEROSCLEROTIC DISTURBANCES

CORONARY ATHEROSCLEROSIS

Coronary artery disease is the leading cause of death in Western society, and the epidemic extends to the rest of the world.

The problem, and at times the drama, of atherosclerotic disease of the coronary arteries stars in a line of cells that form the inner layer of the arteries. This is called the endothelium, and it is present all over the body's arterial tree.

Due to gene influence, poor eating habits, serum lipids abnormalities, diabetes, hypertension, smoking, stress, and other factors, the endothelium becomes damaged, and this results in formation of fatty plaques. Some of these are soft (lipid rich) while others are hard (collagen rich). Both of them may also accumulate calcium.

When the surface of a plaque is injured, it gets damaged in two different ways: it either ruptures or suffers a crack. This leads to the formation of a clot in that particular area (thrombus). The plaque undergoing the process is called a **vulnerable plaque. If the clot is large enough to block the artery completely, the patient may develop a life-threatening arrhythmia, an acute myocardial infarction, or both.**

The majority of heart attacks (myocardial infarctions) originate from atherosclerotic lesions that are not obstructing the coronary artery significantly. A significant coronary obstruction is one that blocks the artery 70 and 80% of its lumen, as seen by a coronary angiogram. A plaque that blocks the lumen of the artery by 50% or less is not considered to be a significantly obstructive lesion since the blood flow going through this obstruction is not affected. Nevertheless, these "mild lesions" are very important in other ways:

- Approximately 80% of acute myocardial infarctions occur with less severe obstructions
- Although a severe blockage is more likely to become occluded by a clot (thrombus) than a lesion with less severe narrowing (stenosis), the less severely narrowed plaques provoke more occlusions. Why?

Because there are many more sites that contain mild to moderate coronary obstructions than critical obstructive lesions

- There is another important factor that renders the atherosclerotic plaque more vulnerable: its softness and lipid content. The larger the lipid pool in the plaque, the greater the plaque's tendency to rupture. A heavily calcified plaque is more resistant to this process. Soft plaques break more easily than the older calcified atherosclerotic plaques

Sometimes, coronary angiograms report that "there are mild, **insignificant** coronary plaques in various coronary arteries."

The way the above should be reported is as follows: "There are no significant *obstructive* coronary lesions." *All* atherosclerotic plaques are significant because they can break and form a clot that blocks the artery acutely and completely.

Conclusion: All atherosclerotic plaque should be treated with respect and great diligence.

The patient with symptoms consistent with acute coronary insufficiency immediately needs a medical environment that will protect him/her. This has to have the capability to do electrocardiographic monitoring and have an available defibrillator.

Ideally, an ECG should be obtained within the first ten minutes. The medical examination priority at this point should be to determine if the patient qualifies for immediate reperfusion therapy (thrombolytic agents, balloon angioplasty) and to provide treatment for life-threatening events.

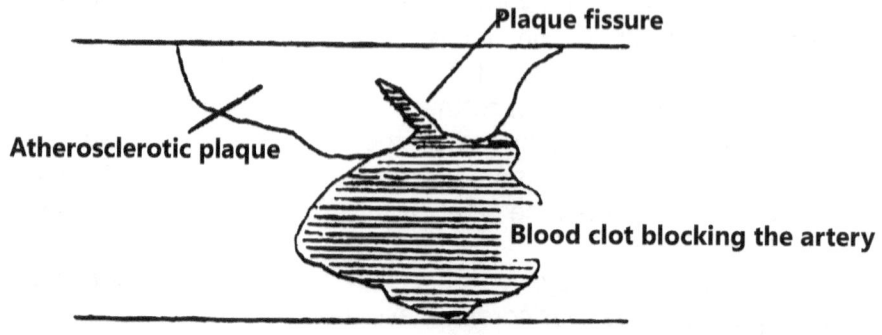

Artery narrowed by a clot that resulted from a fissured plaque

Figure 8

There's some controversy regarding the role of certain infections in the process of plaque vulnerability and their contribution to plaque disruption. *Chlamydia pneumoniae*, herpes viruses, and *Helicobacter pylori*, periodontitis (gum infection), sinusitis, and chronic bronchitis have also been thought by some authors to represent a cause of plaque vulnerability and acute myocardial infarction.

SYMPTOMS OF ACUTE CORONARY INSUFFICIENCY

A reduction of blood supply to the heart muscle due to some obstruction of a coronary artery is called ischemia. Typically, this is expressed by pain or discomfort, usually described as a heaviness, tightness, or constriction in the center of the anterior chest often radiated to the left shoulder and arm. Some patients have no chest discomfort but solely complain of jaw, earlobe, neck, arm, or upper abdominal pain, or shortness of breath.

Acute coronary insufficiency may also present with "atypical" symptoms such as acute shortness of breath, indigestion, unusual location of the pain, agitation, confusion and disorientation, severe weakness, or fainting. Such presentations are more common in women, the elderly, and patients with long-standing diabetes and are associated with higher risk for major complications, death included.

When ischemia (deficient blood supply to the heart muscle) is prolonged, the cardiac muscle gets damaged. That is an acute myocardial infarction. Myocardial infarctions can be silent in about 20% of the cases.

I've seen patients with massive acute myocardial infarctions with no symptoms or minimal symptoms. I once saw a thirty-two-year-old Afro American man, height at 6'7", 270 lbs, with giant muscular development who worked in heavy-duty construction. He complained to the primary physician of "excessive burping," and his ECG was abnormal. He refused hospitalization that day. Three days later I saw him for a consultation at my office and had no complaints. He was feeling "excellent." The reading of his ECG three days prior and on the day of my examination showed a very extensive and acute myocardial infarction. Reluctantly, he accepted to be admitted to the hospital. Still, he kept on saying, "Why should I go to the hospital? There's nothing wrong with me!"

The Chest Pain Evaluation

The evaluation of a patient with chest pain is sometimes difficult, and the diagnosis may be missed, even by experienced doctors. In fact, missing the diagnosis of acute myocardial infarction is the leading cause of malpractice claims for emergency room physicians. To solve this problem, chest pain units adjacent to the ER were developed. Here, the patient is under observation for several hours and is taken several ECG and checked cardiac enzymes to determine if there was myocardial damage.

Risk stratification is done. Those who represent a high risk (markedly positive stress test by nuclear scan or ECG abnormalities at low exercise level) should undergo coronary angiography. Those with negative or low-risk results can be managed medically.

Myocardial ischemia means that the oxygen delivery does not meet the demands of the myocardial muscle. The heart muscle with ischemia is not damaged. Necrosis or infarction (heart muscle damage) develops when ischemia is severe and prolonged.

There are myocardial infarctions of different size: some are small, others quite large, and at times, large enough to be called "massive."

One important factor that determines an infarct's size is the presence (or absence) of collateral circulation.

Collateral circulation results from a chronic severe obstruction of a coronary artery. This leads to other neighboring coronary arteries to develop branches that are normally dormant. These vessels are called collateral vessels and play a great protective role. When a serious

lesion abruptly closes the coronary artery, the collateral circulation prevents the myocardial infarction from happening, or if it happens, it'll be smaller. This is important because infarct size is a significant determinant of survival and congestive heart failure.

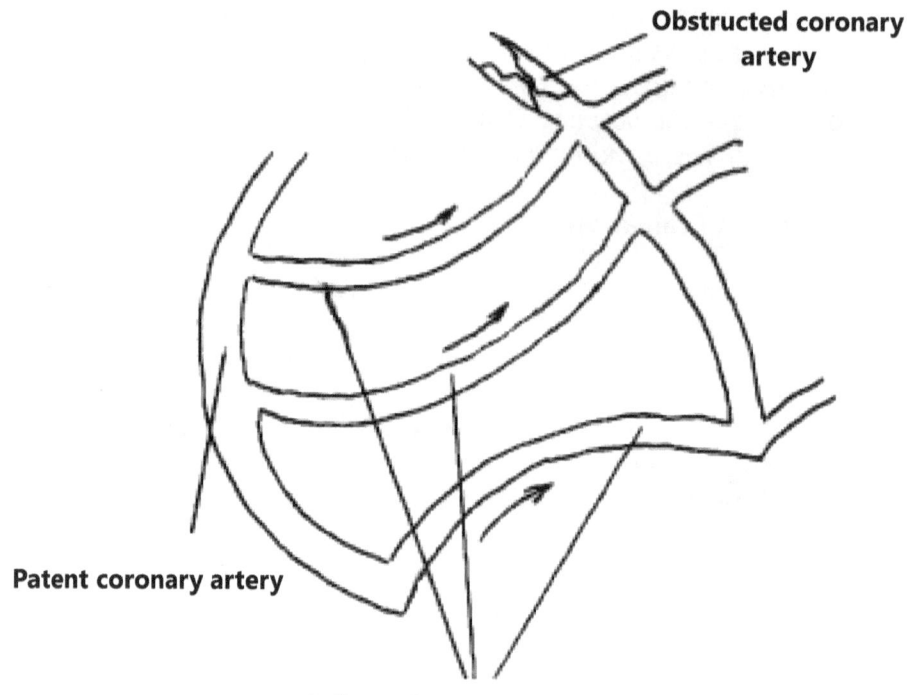

**Obstructed coronary
artery**

Patent coronary artery

**Collateral vessels that supply
blood to the diseased artery**

Collateral circulation

Figure 9

Infarcts that involve 40% or more of the left ventricular (LV) muscle are predictors of cardiogenic shock and death.

Prevention of significant LV damage is attempted by trying to allow the heart muscle to resume the blood flow it needs and, that is, getting it before the coronary artery flow is totally interrupted. Procedures done to restitute a good blood flow are called reperfusion techniques. **Reperfusion then means the return of adequate blood flow through** a coronary artery. The purpose of the reperfusion attempt is damage control and myocardial tissue salvage.

Reperfusion is attempted with clot-dissolving drugs (thrombolytics) and balloon angioplasty. A little balloon is placed in the obstructed region and dilated. When successful, this flattens the plaque and allows an improved or complete resumption of blood flow.

If reperfusion occurs within 4-6 hours following onset of chest pain or ECG changes, there is myocardial salvage. Infarcts that are reperfused after six hours take longer to heal.

Patients who suffer from angina due to coronary atherosclerosis may have a stable pattern: the frequency, severity, location of their chest discomfort is consistent, and they can control the symptoms with appropriate medications. **A change for worse of any of these parameters may be announcing unstable angina**.

There are different degrees of unstable angina. The physician must determine, which cases require careful but not necessarily urgent approach or the need for immediate hospitalization.

ACUTE MYOCARDIAL INFARCTION (AMI) COMPLICATIONS

More than 1.5 million Americans suffer from an acute myocardial infarction annually. In the United States, it is estimated that 13.7 million Americans have coronary heart disease, including more than 7.2 million persons who already have had a myocardial infarction. Patients older than sixty-five years of age carry higher mortality than patients younger than sixty-five years. The major cause of myocardial infarctions is coronary atherosclerosis with an added clot (thrombus), and this mechanism accounts for over 80% of all infarcts. **Other myocardial infarctions are due to non-atherosclerotic diseases of coronary arteries, but they are much less frequent.**

Myocardial cell death occurs 20-30 minutes after occlusion of the artery and is usually complete within 3-6 hours unless timely reperfusion occurs and stops the destructive myocardial process.

If reperfusion occurs within 4-6 hours following onset of chest pain or ECG changes, there is myocardial salvage, and the infarct is likely to affect only the inner layer of the heart called the subendocardial area **(subendocardial infarction).** When the myocardial infarction is extensive and involves the entire thickness of the ventricular wall, it is called **transmural myocardial infarction.**

A subendocardial infarction may be fully healed in 2-3 weeks. Larger infarcts, and those reperfused after six hours, take longer to heal.

Ideally, as previously mentioned, one would like to reperfuse the affected myocardial area within six hours of occlusion to save as much myocardial tissue as possible, **but there appears to be some benefit in opening an artery regardless of the duration of coronary occlusion.**

Sudden death occurs in 25% of patients after an AMI, often before they reach the hospital. Most arrhythmias that are responsible for out-of-hospital sudden coronary deaths are ventricular tachycardia and ventricular fibrillation. The greatest incidence of these rhythms occurs in the first hour.

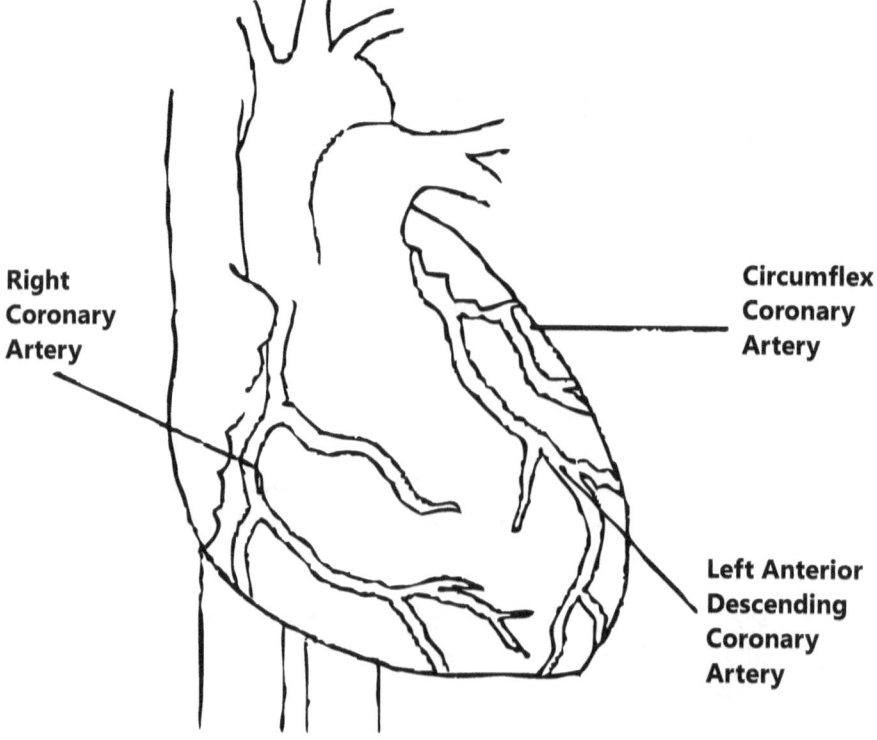

Right Coronary Artery

Circumflex Coronary Artery

Left Anterior Descending Coronary Artery

Normal coronary arteries

Figure 10

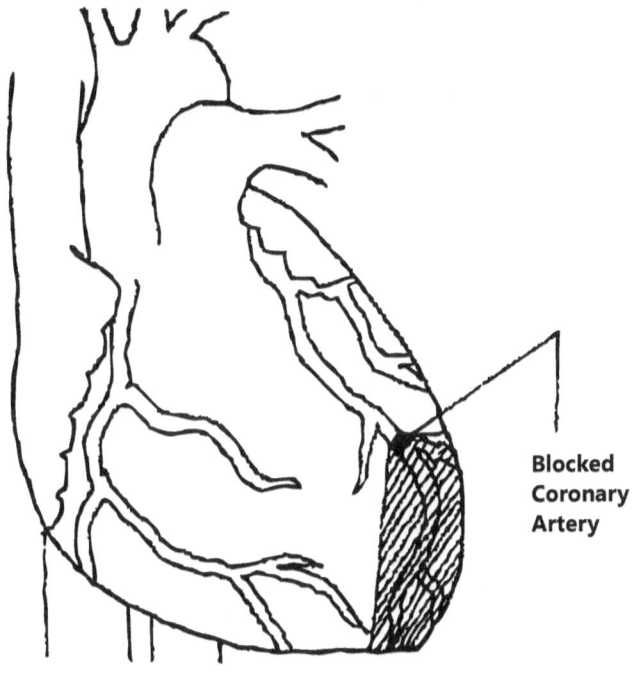

Myocardial infarction

Figure 11

41—CARDIOGENIC SHOCK AND SEVERE HEART FAILURE

Cardiogenic shock is the most common cause of death in patients hospitalized with AMI, and it occurs in 10% of patients who suffer an AMI. The larger the myocardial infarction, the weaker will be the left ventricle. In general, 10% involvement of the left ventricle will minimally reduce the pumping capacity of the heart. On the other hand, severe heart failure and fatal cardiogenic shock is usually associated with involvement of 40% or more of the left ventricular myocardium.

Cardiogenic shock unresponsive to treatment leads to a global cardiovascular collapse: multiple organs do not receive the amount of blood they require to function and that includes the kidneys, the brain, and the rest of the body organs, the heart included.

42—RUPTURE OF INTERVENTRICULAR SEPTUM AND RUPTURE OF A PAPILLARY MUSCLE

These are very acute and life-threatening complications. Treatment varies. It's always complex, and when indicated, a surgical correction is attempted.

Partial rupture of a papillary muscle that normally holds the mitral valve in the right position is a very serious condition, but total rupture of a papillary muscle is incompatible with life because of sudden, massive mitral regurgitation and fulminant heart failure and pulmonary edema.

Cases that are surgically treated have a high mortality rate, but those who survive may do well in the long run.

THE MITRAL VALVE APPARATUS

The mitral valve has two leaflets that are being held by the chordae tendineae. These, in turn, are attached to the papillary muscles which are inserted in the ventricular walls.

Different abnormalities that affect any or various segments of this so-called mitral valve apparatus may cause its malfunction. The repercussions of such disturbances may vary from mild to serious and critical.

Example: Rheumatic fever that affects a child may affect the mitral valve leaflets. The patient recovers from the acute episode of this illness. Twenty-five years later, calcium deposits in the damaged valves and produce a narrowing of the mitral valve opening. (mitral stenosis).

Severe mitral valve prolapse may rupture several chordae tendineae and the valve leaflets are not able to close properly. The valve becomes "insufficient" and regurgitates blood into the left atrium and from here to the lungs causing pulmonary edema or fluid accumulation in both lungs.

An acute myocardial infarction that involves not only the ventricular wall but also a papillary muscle may render the mitral valve insufficient since the papillary muscle has been weakened by "ischemia" or insufficient blood supply due to a blocked coronary artery. In more severe cases, the infarction affecting the papillary muscle produces its rupture with the consequences I just explained in a preceding paragraph.

The following is a basic schematic representation of the normal mitral valve apparatus.

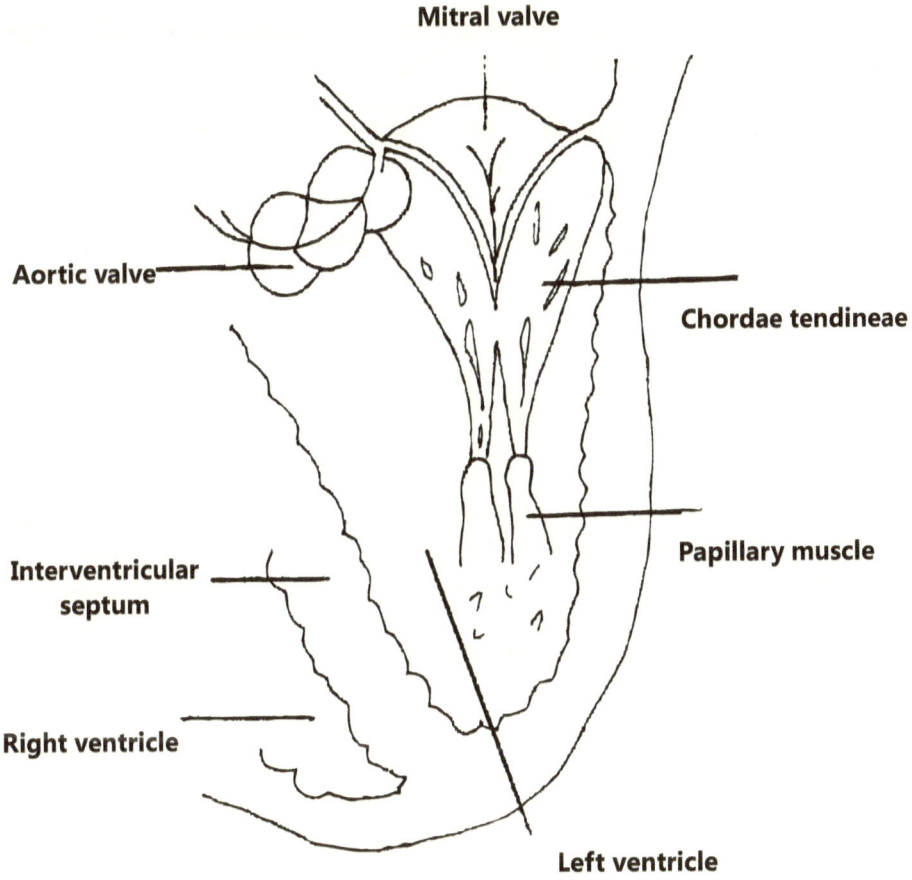

Mitral Valve Apparatus

Figure 12

43—RUPTURE OF THE LEFT VENTRICULAR WALL

The blood fills the pericardial space (pericardial tamponade), and the condition must be dealt with emergently. The incidence of rupture of the left ventricular wall is between 10 and 20%. In contrast, rupture of the ventricular septum is only 2%. Cardiac rupture is seven times more frequent in the left ventricle than in the right ventricle, shows a higher incidence in women, age older than sixty, hypertension and first myocardial infarction, poor collateral circulation, and disease of multiple coronary arteries.

Nearly half of the deaths due to a ruptured myocardial infarction occur before the patient reaches the hospital.

For additional information, please see "**Cardiac Tamponade" (also called pericardial tamponade) at section 98.**

44—CRITICAL CORONARY ARTERY OBSTRUCTION WITHOUT MYOCARDIAL INFARCTION

Some individuals do regular exercises and other physical efforts, and despite of having serious to critical coronary artery blockages, sometimes, amazingly, do not have a myocardial infarction. They develop ventricular fibrillation. Unless they are successfully resuscitated with CPR, they die. This event occurs so fast that there's no time left for the myocardial infarction to take place. This fatal rhythm results from acute lack of oxygen of the cardiac muscle. The myocardium needs blood, and the blocked artery cannot provide it.

Atherosclerotic disease of the coronary arteries is by far the most common cause of their blockages, and in most cases, a clot (thrombus) is present. There are, however, other non-atherosclerotic causes of coronary obstruction (congenital and acquired) that can lead to myocardial infarction and sudden death. These conditions will be described below.

EMBOLISM TO CORONARY ARTERIES

Normal coronary arteries (arteries without plaques) may become acutely blocked and produce an acute myocardial infarction. The typical medical suspicion for this condition is the patient who complains of acute and severe chest pain and has the following:

45—AORTIC AND MITRAL INFECTIVE ENDOCARDITIS OF NATIVE VALVES

Infection of the heart valves creates inflammatory lesions called vegetations. If these affect either the aortic or mitral valve and a tiny fragment breaks off, it moves forward and may enter the opening of a coronary artery causing its blockage and an acute myocardial infarction.

46—PROSTHETIC VALVE ENDOCARDITIS

The risk of prosthetic endocarditis is about 3% in the first year and 0.5% in subsequent years. These infections are difficult to cure, and early reoperation is usually recommended. Careful endocarditis prophylaxis is extraordinarily important. If a tiny clot or a fragment of a vegetation is dislodged from the mitral or aortic prosthesis and enters a coronary artery, a myocardial infarction may ensue.

47—CARDIAC MYXOMAS

Intracardiac myxoma is the most frequent benign tumor of the heart and may develop inside any cardiac chamber although the left atrium is affected in 75% of cases.

Years ago, I witnessed the case of a teenage girl who had a sudden death and her postmortem exam showed a large left atrial (LA) myxoma that had blocked the mitral valve opening. No blood reached the left ventricle and the circulation. That translated into a cardiac arrest. The release of tumor fragments into the general circulation is frequent with this tumor and occurs in 40-50% of patients with LA myxoma. Half of these embolizations involve the brain. Myocardial infarction is occasionally the first manifestation of a myxoma. Surgery is mandatory to excise the myxoma due to the danger of embolization and sudden death.

48—LEFT ATRIAL THROMBUS (CLOT)

Clots characteristically develop in the left atrium as a result of a dilated cardiomyopathy, when the heart muscle becomes weak and flabby. This predisposes to clot formation. Mitral stenosis, usually due to rheumatic fever (in elderly people, heavy calcification of the mitral valve can do it), narrows the opening of the mitral valve. This increases the pressure inside the left atrium and enlarges this chamber. This may result in clot or thrombus formation

A cardiac arrhythmia, atrial fibrillation, causes the left atrium to contract weakly and irregularly, also predisposes to clot formation inside that cardiac chamber and that is the reason why patients with this arrhythmia are often medicated with the anticoagulant warfarin.

49—LEFT VENTRICULAR THROMBUS (CLOT)

Acute myocardial infarctions may produce a clot in the wall of the damaged left ventricle. This usually occurs within the first three days or weeks following the acute myocardial infarction. This phenomenon is unlikely to develop after 4-6 weeks. Anticoagulation is useful to reduce the incidence of thrombus formation.

Cardiomyopathies also have a propensity to form intracavitary ventricular clots. A cardiac ultrasound usually detects these clots.

Once the clot fragments are released, the damage they cause depends upon their destination. If they enter a coronary artery, an acute MI occurs. If they penetrate the spleen, the patient will have acute left upper quadrant pain. If the clots choose the brain as the landing place, a stroke will follow. If the clots moves south toward the arteries of the groin or the leg, the leg and foot will become acutely pale and painful.

50—CORONARY ARTERY BLOCKAGE DUE TO HEMATOLOGICAL (BLOOD) DISORDERS

Patients with normal coronary arteries who suffer from hematological disease may have acute myocardial infarctions, arrhythmias, and sudden death when large quantities of abnormal cells form plugs that block the lumen of the coronary artery. Examples include the following: leukemia (blood cancer), polycythemia vera (abnormally large number of red blood cells), sickle cell anemia (hereditary condition that has abundant blood sickle cells), and primary thrombocytosis (excessive number of platelets).

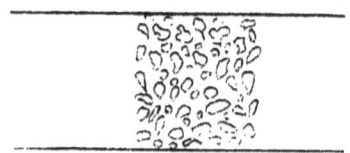

Dense concentration of abnormal blood cells

Figure 13

51—CORONARY ARTERY BLOCKAGE WITH "NORMAL" CORONARY ARTERIES—SPONTANEOUS OR COCAINE-INDUCED CORONARY ARTERY SPASM

Coronary artery spasm that significantly narrows the lumen (inner diameter) of the vessel has been associated with chest pains (angina), acute myocardial infarction, and sudden death.

It seems that the muscular layer of the artery constrict in response to various emotional reactions as well as some circulating substances in the blood, such as catecholamines, thromboxane, and prostaglandins.

Three newly recognized provocative factors that cause coronary spasm and acute myocardial infarction includes general anesthesia, "allergic angina" (histamine-induced, and in women postpartum receiving bromocriptine in the presence of pregnancy-induced hypertension).

Pheochromocytomas (adrenal gland tumors) that produce excessive amounts of catecholamines are capable of causing coronary spasms.

It isn't clear why sometimes normal-appearing coronary arteries constrict spontaneously.

I've seen a number of these cases, but two of them impressed so much that I'll never forget them: one was the case of a woman of high socioeconomic status in her fifties, who was arrested by the police "unfairly" and was accused of stealing a 10 cents pen at a store. She was placed behind bars for several hours until her husband got her release on bail. That night she had a massive acute myocardial infarction and proven normal coronary arteries by angiogram. The severe stress she went through was thought to cause prolonged spasm of a major coronary artery. Her coronary angiogram showed "normal" coronary arteries.

**

Another case occurred several decades ago: an Afro American gentleman of fifty-two years of age had multiple episodes of ventricular fibrillation with angiographically normal coronary arteries. While in the hospital, he developed multiple episodes of ventricular fibrillation (proven by monitor), and I succeeded in changing that lethal rhythm with a thump in his chest, over his heart. This is not a usually effective or recommendable technique to correct ventricular fibrillation, but in this case, it worked wonders. Those days, a drug called nifedipine had not been approved by the FDA. The Miami Heart Institute was running a research project with that drug. I was permitted to use it, gave it to the patient, and the results were magic. No more spasms . . . none for a few months. Then, the patient was lost for follow-up.

Cocaine abuse is a major social-medical problem: More than 22 million Americans have tried cocaine at least once, and 5 million are currently using it. This substance causes coronary vasoconstriction and myocardial infarctions in the absence of coronary artery disease. Cocaine-induced coronary vasoconstriction has been reported in patients following the intranasal administration of cocaine.

The coronary spasm may end in sudden death. Massive cocaine-induced production of norepinephrine has a lot to do with the artery constriction.

Besides the coronary spasms, sometimes cocaine has produced intravascular clots responsible for the heart attack. The inner layer of the artery is damaged, and there's also platelet aggregation with a propensity to clot formation.

Excessive administration of vasoconstrictors by the use of nose drops containing phenylephrine may also cause vasospasm and myocardial infarction (see section 39).

There are two drugs being considered as possible causes for coronary spasms and lethal arrhythmias: MDMA or ectasy, and MDEA or eve.

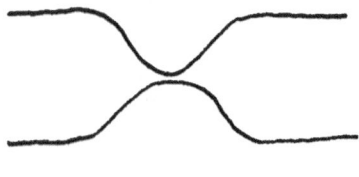

Coronary artery spasm

Figure 14

CORONARY ARTERY BLOCKAGE DUE TO THICKENING OF THE ARTERIAL WALL

52—PSEUDOXANTOMA ELASTICUM

This is a rare heritable disorder characterized by the progressive accumulation of mineral substances within the elastic fibers of arteries involving the cardiovascular system, skin, brain, and gastrointestinal tract. The arteries also have abundant calcium deposits. This disease is associated with higher incidence of coronary artery disease.

53—RADIATION THERAPY

Accelerated or premature atherosclerosis has been increasingly reported in the medical literature in young individuals treated with radiation to the thorax for various malignancies. The incidence varies from 0.13 to 2.7% who receive this kind of treatment. Some of these patients developed angina or myocardial infarctions and were treated with angioplasty or coronary bypass surgery. The scars produced by radiation therapy may present greater than average difficulties to negotiate the narrowed coronary arteries by balloon angioplasty. Sometimes, coronary disease due to radiation appears 5-10 years following radiation.

Chemotherapy-induced myocardial infarction in a young man has been reported too. Vascular toxicity, including myocardial infarction, has been reported following anticancer regimen containing Vinca alkaloids.

Thickening of the arterial wall

Figure 15

54—CORONARY ARTERY OBSTRUCTION DUE TO METABOLIC DISORDER

These are inborn errors of metabolism. **Deposition of abnormal material may severely narrow the coronary artery lumen and produce an acute myocardial infarction or sudden death (mucopolysaccharidoses, oxalosis, homocystinuria, and others).**

Specific metabolic substances accumulate in the walls of large and small coronary arteries.

Patients suffering from thoracic cancers may have additional problems, such as cardiac invasion by the tumor, marked blood coagulability, and coronary artery spasms.

CONGENITAL ANOMALIES OF CORONARY ARTERIES

55—ANOMALOUS TAKEOFF OF A CORONARY ARTERY

Congenital coronary artery anomalies are found in approximately 1% of all patients undergoing angiography and 0.3% of patients undergoing autopsy. In about 30% of these cases, SCD has occurred and has usually been exercise-induced.

Origin of the left main coronary artery from the right aortic sinus or origin of the right coronary artery from the left coronary sinus, are the variants most frequently associated with SCD.

The diagnosis is considered in children with chest pains or myocardial infarctions. Sometimes they have a heart murmur and an abnormal ECG.

56—CORONARY FISTULA

This is an abnormal communication between a major coronary artery and a cardiac chamber, a major vessel (vena cava, pulmonary artery), or other vascular structure. It is an infrequent abnormality. It can affect any age. Many coronary fistulas are small and produce no symptoms, whereas others are large enough to produce a loud murmur, angina, myocardial infarction, heart failure, and SCD. Treatment is surgical for patients with symptoms or those asymptomatic patients who are candidates for further complications.

57—ATROPHIC CORONARY ARTERIES

Sometimes, the coronary arteries do not develop and become atrophic. The medical term to define this condition is *atresia*. This abnormality is capable of causing a heart attack with all the risks that this implies. The area of the heart affected becomes dependent on collateral coronary blood flow, which originates in a neighboring coronary vessel.

58—CORONARY ARTERY DISSECTION

Coronary arteries have three layers: the intima, which is in direct contact with the circulating blood, the media, and the external layer also called adventitia. Separation of the media by hemorrhage is termed *coronary artery dissection*.

This condition may be an extension of an aortic root aneurysm, a result from coronary angioplasty or angiography, cardiac surgery, or chest trauma.

Sometimes, coronary artery dissection is spontaneous and occur in women who are most commonly postpartum. This may result in sudden death or acute myocardial infarction and subsequent death.

INFLAMMATION OF THE CORONARY ARTERIES—NONINFECTIOUS ANGIITIS

There are numerous diseases that can cause inflammation of the coronary arteries. I'll just describe a few below.

59—PERIARTERITIS NODOSA (PA)

This is a chronic disease associated with coronary angiitis, infarctions or hemorrhages in various organs. Cardiac complications also occur as a result of the chronic hypertension that occurs in 90% of patients with PA.

60—KAWASAKI DISEASE

This is a disease that affects children. It's an acute febrile illness associated with inflamed lymph nodes and a rash. The disease was first described in Japan in 1967 but subsequently it was reported all over the world in all racial groups. Arteries are diffusely inflamed, and coronary arteries form aneurysms in 25% of cases. When small, sometimes the aneurysms regress, particularly in children under one year of age. Coronary arteries may become occluded, resulting in myocardial infarction and sudden death.

COLLAGEN VASCULAR DISEASES—VASCULITIS

These involve arthritis, myositis (inflammation of muscles), carditis (inflammation of heart muscle and valves), and dermatitis. Typical examples include **rheumatoid arthritis associated with rheumatoid arteritis, temporal arteritis, Takayasu arteritis, systemic lupus erythematosus (SLE).**

61—RHEUMATOID ARTHRITIS

This **is the most common of the connective tissue diseases** and is characterized by its deforming erosions of the joints. This disease is associated with higher incidence of myocardial infarctions and strokes and higher cardiovascular mortality. Atherosclerosis appears to occur at an accelerated rate.

62—TEMPORAL ARTERITIS

This is a diffuse vascular inflammation that affects multiple arteries. It is also called giant cell arteritis. It occurs almost exclusively in patients older than fifty-five years of age. Common symptoms are headaches, visual disturbances, anemia, and in 50% of patients, polymyalgia rheumatica with diffuse muscular pains.

63—TAKAYASU ARTERITIS (PULSELESS DISEASE)

This is a chronic inflammatory vascular disease that can end abruptly with an acute myocardial infarction. Its origin is unknown. It has a worldwide distribution, but it is more frequent in young to middle-aged women. **Any young woman who presents with an acute myocardial infarction should be suspected of having Takayasu's disease.**

64—SYSTEMIC LUPUS ERYTHEMATOSUS

This affects all races, but the disease is usually more severe in blacks than in whites, and it is also more frequent in females. Female to male ratio is 8:1.

The disease affects multiple tissues and organs, and it is usually chronic although it may have an acute, fulminating course with an acute myocardial infarction and even sudden death sometimes, not associated with an acute myocardial infarction.

65—CORONARY ARTERY ALLERGIC VASCULITIS

This is an allergic reaction that affects the coronary arteries and it's caused by various drugs. The most common medications associated with this phenomenon are penicillin, methyldopa, sulfas, tetracycline, and the drugs to treat tuberculosis. The trouble with this kind of allergy is that it often goes unnoticed, and the first expression of the disease may be sudden death due to a cardiac arrhythmia.

There are a number of conditions that cause an allergic reaction inside the coronary arteries that are capable of blocking them. Organ-transplantation arteritis is a typical example. It's a form of immune-mediated vascular injury.

66—INFECTIONS OF THE CORONARY ARTERIES— INFECTIOUS ANGIITIS

Some examples include the following: endocarditis, syphilis, malaria, viruses, rickettsial infections, typhus, leprosy, tuberculosis, salmonella.

67—CORONARY ARTERY TRAUMA

Coronary arteries may be injured by non-penetrating blunt chest wall injury such as a steering wheel or penetrating trauma such as a laceration from a stab wound or bullet. An accidental injury may occur during coronary bypass surgery or with coronary angiography or angioplasty. Non-penetrating trauma may produce coronary injury resulting in coronary dissection, contusion, clot formation (thrombosis), fistula, and coronary artery aneurysm formation.

Curiously, extensive coronary artery dissections occur more commonly as the result of catheter injury in normal coronary arteries than in coronary arteries with severe atherosclerotic plaques.

68—MYOCARDIAL OXYGEN DEMAND-SUPPLY IMBALANCE

Sometimes, the coronary arteries may be completely normal, but the blood they carry does not transport the right amount of oxygen to all tissues and organs. Oxygen is vital for organs to function properly. A typical example of deficient oxygen supply is the intoxication by carbon monoxide, which means poor delivery of oxygen.

During a thyroid storm, the oxygen supply side is not affected, but the need of the myocardium for oxygen greatly increases due to the hypermetabolic needs resulting from the hyperthyroid state (tachycardia and stronger cardiac contractions). The result is an oxygen deficiency that may lead to myocardial infarction and/or lethal arrhythmias.

DISEASE OF THE CARDIAC MUSCLE—CARDIOMYOPATHIES

Cardiomyopathy is a primary disorder of the heart muscle that impairs the cardiac function and **is not caused by disease of any other cardiac structures.** Let me clarify this concept: The cardiac muscle may be weakened by disease of the coronary arteries or cardiac valves, congenital heart disease or an injury, but sometimes, the problem is a process that **primarily affected the cardiac muscle. In other words, from all of the structures existing in the heart anatomy, the cardiac muscle is the one that is affected first.**

There are different kinds of cardiomyopathies: some dilate the cavities of the heart, others produce a thick heart muscle, another group makes the heart stiff. **There are then three fundamentally different types of cardiomyopathies (dilated, hypertrophic, and restrictive).**

Each of these categories is produced by a number of different provocative factors. Their severity shows great variations too. Some of them improve to the point where patients are able to return to working activities and have a normal life, and their hearts go back to normal. Others suffer a chronic course with some discomforts (fatigue, shortness of breath, chest heaviness, palpitations, edema). The cardiac function remains impaired, but the patient lives with his/her cardiac disease fairly well although with some physical restrictions and limitations. Those less fortunate develop a severe form of cardiomyopathy that leads to total disability with chronic congestive heart failure, life-threatening arrhythmias, and the possibility of sudden death. Sometimes, a heart transplant is the best option, but, for different reasons, not all patients with severe cardiomyopathy can be treated that way.

- *Dilated cardiomyopathies.* The left ventricle is dilated, and its pumping action is weakened (systolic dysfunction).
- *Hypertrophic cardiomyopathies.* The left ventricle is thick without obstruction to the ejection of blood from the left ventricle (**hypertrophic non-obstructive cardiomyopathy**), or the ventricles are thick and the upper septum is prominent and obstructs the ejection of blood from the left ventricle (**hypertrophic obstructive cardiomyopathy**)
- *Restrictive cardiomyopathies.* This group offers resistance to the filling of the left ventricle, and this is called diastolic dysfunction.

The causes of these various cardiomyopathies capable of causing a rapid or sudden death are so numerous that it cannot be mentioned, let alone described, in this book.

DILATED CARDIOMYOPATHY (dilated cardiac cavities and weak heart muscle)

69—IDIOPATHIC DILATED CARDIOMYOPATHY (IDC), INCLUDING FAMILIAL FORMS

In a way, this disease is an enigma. On the least expected day, the patient feels severe fatigue, shortness of breath, and swollen legs due to fluid accumulation. Both ventricles appear dilated and weak, and the cause of the disorder is totally unknown. In the last few years, there have been familial cases of this illness, and gene mutations were felt to be responsible for the dilatation and poor function of the ventricles. The clinical presentation is not different than a viral myocarditis, an alcoholic cardiomyopathy, or hypo—or hyperthyroidism. When none of these and a long list of provocative agents capable of causing a dilated cardiomyopathy are reasonably excluded, then the diagnosis of idiopathic dilated cardiomyopathy is established. *Idiopathic* means a disease of unknown origin.

DCM may be familial in as many as 35-50% of the cases when first-degree relatives are closely screened. Many genetic mutations are the cause of these familial DCM.

Some cases recover, and others are prone to a sudden death due to arrhythmias.

A few years ago, the survival was approximately 50% in five years. Therapy of this condition has greatly improved this condition's outlook. Various drugs, special pacemakers, implantable cardiac defibrillator, and in some cases, heart transplantation offer a much better outcome.

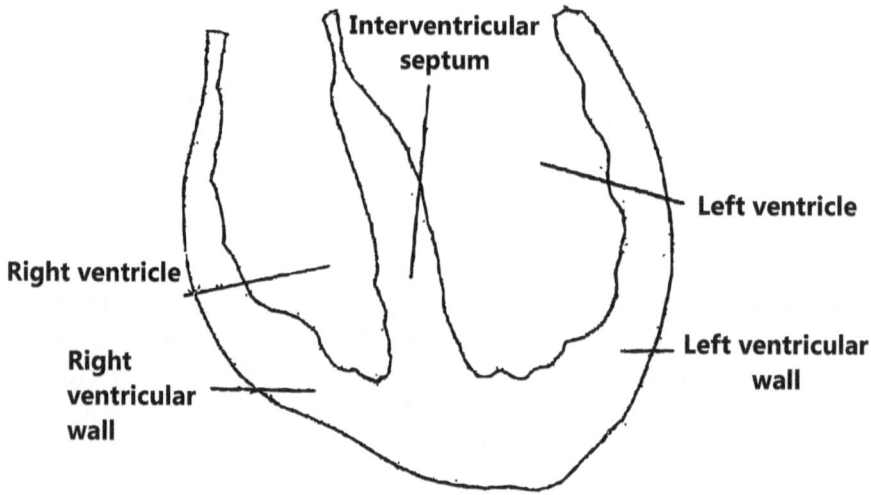

Normal heart
Interventricular septum, right and left ventricular
walls and cavities

Figure 16

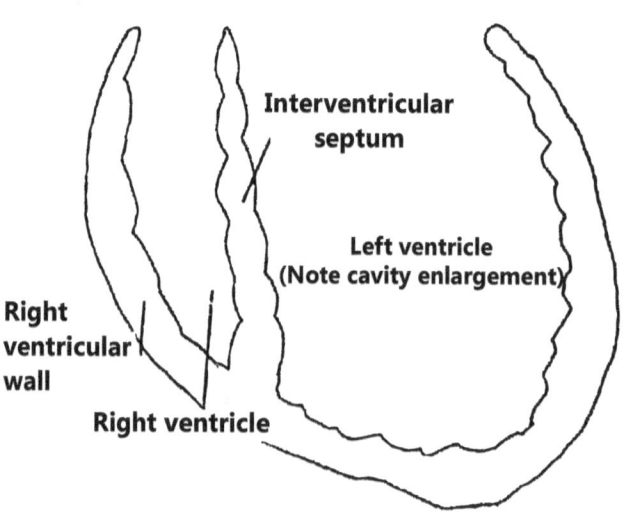

Dilated cardiomyopathy

Figure 17

70—ALCOHOLIC CARDIOMYOPATHY

This diagnosis is established when other causes of heart failure have been excluded and there is a history of chronic alcohol abuse. The required amount of alcohol consumption to produce an alcoholic cardiomyopathy is in excess of 80 g of alcohol per day for males and 40 g of alcohol for women for more than five years. Some individuals, however, are more susceptible, and lower amounts of alcohol cause the disease as well. Chronic alcohol abuse accounts for up to 45% of all dilated cardiomyopathies. In one study, 20% of chronic alcoholic women and 26% of chronic alcoholic men in a five-year period develop dilated cardiomyopathy.

Chronic alcohol consumption may result in hypertension, heart failure, and life-threatening arrhythmias.

Sudden death can be the initial presentation of alcoholic cardiomyopathy.

These patients are not usually candidates for cardiac transplantation because of the high relapse rate of alcoholism.

71—HYPERTENSIVE CARDIOMYOPATHY

This is the result of long-standing hypertension. To attribute this cardiomyopathy to hypertension, it is estimated that this has been uncontrolled, high (>160/100 mmHg), and sustained for years.

72—VALVULAR CARDIOMYOPATHY

A dilated cardiomyopathy most commonly occurs when there's severe leakage (regurgitation) of the aortic or mitral valve, less commonly with aortic stenosis. The left ventricle becomes enlarged due to the increased stress on its walls.

73—HYPOTHYROIDISM

Hypothyroidism is a frequent disorder, and occasionally, the diagnosis is missed. Even advanced hypothyroidism may not be suspected. I remember the cases of two elderly women who were in coma, and I was called in consultation because they had life-threatening arrhythmias. Both of them happened to be in myxedema coma, an expression of very severe, unrecognized, untreated hypothyroidism. Both recovered.

These patients needed, among other things, the correction of the thyroid hormone deficiency.

74—THYROID STORM AND CARDIOVASCULAR COLLAPSE

The extreme opposite of coma due to hypothyroidism is a thyroid storm. This is an acute and very serious complication of Graves' disease or hyperthyroidism that got out of control.

The thyroid storm is a dreaded condition. The patient is febrile, profoundly weak, extremely restless, confused or psychotic, and may even go into coma. All of the above is associated with cardiovascular collapse and shock. Most of these patients have neck masses due to goiter. Mortality of a thyroid storm used to be 20% years back. Current medical advances in treating this condition have significantly improved its outlook. The thyroid gland is located in the neck and produces thyroid hormone. This hormone is essential for the normal function of body cells. When there's an excess of it, the condition is called hyperthyroidism. When the thyroid hormone levels are too high, a thyroid storm is imminent. This is a dire emergency. The disorder can be fatal.

One clinical feature that distinguishes hyperthyroidism from a thyroid storm is the body temperature. The latter reaches temperatures as high as 105-106 °F.

WHAT PRECIPITATES A THYROID STORM?

- Infection
- Thyroid surgery in a hyperthyroid patient
- Stopping medications for hyperthyroidism
- Too high dose of thyroid hormone
- Treatment with radioactive iodine
- Pregnancy
- Acute myocardial infarction or other cardiac emergencies

SYMPTOMS

Any patient diagnosed with hyperthyroidism that develops one or more of the following symptoms should be transported to an ED immediately:

- Tachycardia
- Shortness of breath or chest pains

- Anxiety
- Severe weakness
- Excessive perspiration
- Heart failure

TREATMENT

- Fever control
- Sometimes oxygen
- Intravenous steroids
- To block the action of thyroid hormone on cells, a beta-blocker such as propranolol is used
- Iodide to block the thyroid hormone release
- Propylthiouracil (PTU) or methimazole to block production of thyroid hormone

PREVENTION

Early treatment of hyperthyroidism

HELPFUL LINKS

American Thyroid Association
Thyroid Foundation of America
America Foundation of Thyroid Patients

75—PHEOCHROMOCYTHOMA

This is an adrenal gland tumor that manufactures toxic amounts of catecholamines. These lead to a cardiomyopathy. When the presentation of the tumor is aggressive, patients tend to die of cardiac complications, typically acute heart failure or deadly arrhythmias. Emergent treatment with alpha and beta-blockers and prompt adrenalectomy (resection of the adrenal gland that contains the tumor) can be lifesaving, and the cardiac abnormalities can be reversed.

76—ACROMEGALY

This disease is produced by a pituitary gland tumor that produces excessive growth hormone.

Ten to twenty percent of patients with this condition develop heart failure. The heart is infiltrated with excessive collagen tissue, and this replaces part of the heart muscle. This makes the acromegalic heart highly resistant to the treatment of heart failure. Furthermore, the collagen spreads like a spiderweb, involving the conducting or electrical system of the heart that may be responsible for arrhythmias capable of causing sudden death.

77—ISCHEMIC CARDIOMYOPATHY

This condition results from previous myocardial infarctions that have significantly and permanently damaged the left ventricle, sometimes up to 50% of the left ventricular mass, or have shown evidence of significant obstruction of a major coronary artery of 70% or more. The left ventricular function is severely impaired, and the ejection fraction, the marker expression of the left ventricular strength, is low, usually 30-35% and occasionally 10-15%. An average of about one-fourth of the patients who sustained a myocardial infarction in the anterior wall of the left ventricle dilated this chamber 12-24 months after the heart attack. Treatment is provided with digitalis, ACE inhibitors, beta-blockers, spironolactone, diuretics, and at times, anticoagulants to prevent formation of clots in a very poorly functioning left ventricle, pacemakers, and implantation of a cardiac defibrillator to prevent a sudden death.

78—PERIPARTUM CARDIOMYOPATHY

She was twenty-five years of age, African American, and had delivered a normal baby a month prior. One morning, she walked up with extreme fatigue, swelling of her legs, and shortness of breath. She saw me the same in the afternoon hours. She had congestive heart failure, chest x-ray showed a huge heart shadow, her echocardiogram documented extremely poor function of the cardiac pump. After several months of treatment, the heart remained very weak, and she was referred for cardiac transplantation.

What I just described is the so-called peripartum cardiomyopathy, a weak heart that appears during the last month of pregnancy or within five months after delivery. The cause of this illness is unknown. The heart size is markedly enlarged. In the United States, this condition appears 1 in every 1,300-4,000 deliveries, and although it appears at any age, it's more common after age thirty, African Americans, multiple pregnancies, alcoholism, and malnutrition. Treatment includes absolute prohibition of smoking and drinking, salt restriction, diuretics, digitalis, ACE inhibitors, a beta-blocker, and other measures used to deal with advanced congestive heart failure. The disease carries a death rate of 25-50%. Some women react favorably, and their heart size returns to normal soon following delivery. This is a very good sign, and recovery is possible. Others suffer from heart failure but remain stable for some time while others, like the patient I described, continue to have a very weak heart or get even worse in a short period of time. These are the cases that may require a heart transplant.

Women who survive the disease should avoid future pregnancies and discuss with the physician methods of contraception.

79—INFECTIOUS CARDIOMYOPATHY

Viral, bacterial, rickettsial, protozoal, parasitic, and fungal myocarditis. Any of these agents may cause a dilated cardiomyopathy.

Sometimes, viral myocarditis, like viral hepatitis, may be transient and be unrecognized by the patient and the doctor. A flu virus, for example, may affect the heart, and the patient's only physical evidence for it is an acceleration of the heartbeat, which is a suspicious sign when the patient is not having a temperature elevation. After a few days, the patient's flu is gone and so is the myocarditis. This "touched" the heart but caused no permanent damage.

The possibility that the heart might be involved during a flu infection should always be kept in mind. Those suffering from a viral infection should refrain from doing any physical exercises until they are fully recovered. An athlete running a marathon in Boston years back had the flu and decided to compete anyway. He collapsed and died, and a postmortem examination showed an acute viral myocarditis. There's a good chance that nothing serious would had happened to him if he had kept bed rest.

TOXIC CARDIOMYOPATHIES

Chemotherapeutic agents are drugs used to treat cancer. Some of them can cause acute or chronic cardiomyopathy. The most common anticancer agents associated with heart failure are the **anthracycline group (doxorubicin) and cyclophosphamide.**

80—ANTRACYCLINE-INDUCED CARDIOMYOPATHY

The anthracycline antibiotic anticancer drugs, doxorubicin and daunorubicin, lead to a dose-related cardiomyopathy, and the heart muscle is affected with cumulative doses. In fact, the incidence of heart failure dramatically increases when the cumulative doses of 450 mg/m^2 have been given to patients who had no previous evidence of heart disease. Doxorubicin has been used as a single agent or in combination with other drugs for the treatment of breast and esophageal cancer as well as sarcomas and lymphomas.

Risk factors for the development of doxorubicin cardiomyopathy include age older than seventy years, combination therapy with cyclophosphamide or paclitaxel, previous mediastinal irradiation, prior heart disease, hypertension, and liver disease. Cardiac toxicity may become evident within a year of the last dose of anthracycline or as late as twenty years after the last administered dose.

The outlook and prognosis of the anthracycline cardiomyopathy is poor. The prognosis is better when the cardiomyopathy appears months to years after administration of this agent.

Cyclophosphamide, at times, can be lethal too. However, those who survive and recover experience no residual cardiac damage.

Treatment for heart failure must be aggressive since some patients improve considerably with it.

81—NUTRITIONAL DEFICIENCIES AND SOME OTHER TOXIC AGENTS THAT MAY CAUSE CARDIOMYOPATHY

Nutritional deficiencies due to thiamine (Vitamin B1), selenium, carnitine, and protein may lead to dilatation and weakness of the heart muscle. These are prevalent in underdeveloped societies.

Amphetamines, antidepressants, antiretroviral agents (drugs to treat HIV such as zidovudine, didanosine, zalcitabine) catecholamines, arsenic, lithium, interferon, cobalt, scorpions, snakes, spiders, and many others can produce myocarditis and serious cardiac arrhythmias.

An increased incidence of cardiomyopathy has been recently reported with a psychotropic drug use to treat schizophrenia called **clozapine.** All cardiac chambers were noted to be dilated, but the process may recede by discontinuation of the drug. The duration of treatment with this drug prior to the development of cardiomyopathy ranges from two weeks to seven years with a median duration of nine months. Of the 178 cases reported by the drug manufacturer, 18% were fatal.

82—ACUTE ALCOHOLIC INTOXICATION

Alcohol irritates the stomach, and when drank in excess, it induces vomiting. The breathing and gag reflex are impaired in alcoholic intoxication. A person who is not conscious may aspirate gastric contents and die from asphyxiation.

Remember that a person's blood alcohol concentration (BAC) can continue to rise even after he or she stops drinking since there's alcohol in the stomach and intestines that continues to be absorbed and circulates in the bloodstream.

SIGNS OF ALCOHOL POISONING

- Mental confusion, stupor, coma
- Vomiting
- Seizures (resulting from alcohol-induced hypoglycemia)
- Slow breathing (fewer than eight breaths per minute)
- No breathing for ten seconds or more between breaths
- Low body temperature
- Pale, bluish skin

Left untreated or treated with delay, alcohol poisoning may lead to permanent brain damage and sudden or rapid death. This results from acute heart failure, severe arrhythmias, or a combination of both.

CARDIOMYOPATHY DUE TO IMMUNE REACTION

83—ACUTE RHEUMATIC FEVER AND ACUTE RHEUMATIC CARDITIS

Acute rheumatic fever (ARF) is a disease that involves many organs and systems of the human body. It is an autoimmune disease that results from infection with group A *Streptococcus*. Unless preventive measures are taken, the disease tends to recur, and the more times it does that, the greater the chances that it will leave permanent damage in the cardiac valves.

ARF is currently uncommon in developed countries but remains a serious health problem in underdeveloped societies and also in poor or indigenous populations of wealthy countries.

Death from ARF is rare during the acute period of the disease. When it occurs, it's due to acute inflammation of the myocardium, the so-called rheumatic carditis. This can result in severe heart failure and lethal arrhythmias.

84—SARCOIDOSIS

This is a disease of unknown origin characterized by deposits of lesions in different organs called granulomas. Lung, liver, spleen, lymph nodes, skin are involved. Granulomas involve the heart in as many as 25% of patients. Some patients (and the doctors who treat them) may not be aware of the cardiac involvement, but in half of the fatalities in sarcoidosis, the heart was responsible for the demise. Echocardiogram and MRI may help to discover the cardiac involvement. Usually, the cardiac diagnosis is based upon abnormalities present in these tests plus the positive biopsies obtained from organs (e.g., liver, lymph node, or skin) more easily accessible than the heart. There's no specific treatment for this disorder, but some people require permanent pacemaker or an implantable intracardiac defibrillator to prevent sudden cardiac death.

85—CHAGAS CARDIOMYOPATHY

Dr. Chagas was an Argentine investigator who worked at the University of Buenos Aires, Infectious Diseases, Muniz Hospital at a time when I was also working at the same institution. He used to walk alone toward his laboratory. I used to say to him, with reverential respect: "Buenos dias, Dr. Chagas." He kindly responded, "Buenos dias, hijo." His research on this disease made him immortal.

Chagas disease is the most common cause of non-atherosclerotic cardiomyopathy in South and Central America, with over 10 million people affected. It is caused by a parasite called *Tripanosoma cruzi*. The vector is a bug known in Spanish as *vinchuca*. The basis for the cardiomyopathy is unknown but may be immunologic. Severe cases of Chagas myocarditis can be fatal. There's no specific treatment for this disease, but pacemakers, intracardiac defibrillators, and treatment for heart failure may be lifesaving.

86—REJECTION OF A TRANSPLANTED HEART

The transplanted heart may be rejected by the recipient. The rejection may be acute, superacute, and chronic.

Hyperacute rejections manifests as severe graft failure within the first few minutes to hours after transplantation. There is fever, heart failure, or low blood pressure (hypotension).

Predisposing factors include presensitization following multiple previous blood transfusions or multiple pregnancies. Without mechanical circulatory support and emergent retransplantation, the patient usually does not survive.

87—HYPERTROPHIC CARDIOMYOPATHY (THICK MUSCLE)

Left ventricular hypertrophy (LVH) has been identified as a strong factor for sudden death. LVH can be seen in association with chronic blockage of coronary arteries, hypertension, disease of the cardiac valves, advanced age (here, many cardiac cells becomes atrophic and the remaining cardiac muscle cells become larger [hypertrophied] to compensate for the former's deficient function) and morbid obesity.

A thick left ventricle predisposes to dangerous ventricular arrhythmias: the coronary arteries running inside the heart muscle get partly squeezed, and this results in decreased blood flow to the heart muscle (ischemia). This, in turn, leads to myocardial cells scarring (fibrosis) and predisposes to life-threatening arrhythmias.

88—HYPERTROPHIC OBSTRUCTIVE CARDIOMYOPATHY (HOCM)

This is an inheritable disease of the heart muscle. Its prevalence is 1:500 to 1:1,000 persons. It is an unpredictable and capricious disorder. At times, patients suffer from fainting attacks (syncope), chest pains, and shortness of breath while others have no symptoms whatsoever throughout the course of their lives. HOCM is the most common cause of sudden cardiac death in young people, including athletes. Treatment approach varies from case to case.

In HOCM the heart muscle becomes thick, but with one notable characteristic. The upper part of the septum becomes so thick that when it contracts forcefully, it blocks the exit of blood from the left ventricle into the general circulation. The result is a temporary cutoff of blood supply to the brain. The patient collapses. At times recovery follows, but other times, ventricular fibrillation and death occur.

The ventricles are not only thick but stiff, which causes shortness of breath. That thick muscle also compresses the branches of the coronary arteries that run their course inside that muscle, and this causes myocardial ischemia (decreased blood supply to the heart muscle) and myocardial infarctions (damage to the heart muscle). The abnormally thick muscle distorts the mitral valve apparatus. This results in mitral valve regurgitation.

The disease may be discovered by a routine abnormal electrocardiogram: most patients show left ventricular hypertrophy, which means a thick, enlarged left ventricle; a heart murmur; or a screening echocardiogram.

Sudden death is most frequent in young adults but may also occur in the elderly. It may also occur in those who never had any symptoms. This has been observed mostly following intense physical activities. Thus, young athletes with HOCM should not engage in competitive sports. Death results from an arrhythmia: VT or ventricular tachycardia followed by VF or ventricular fibrillation.

These patients should be carefully watched for endocarditis and atrial fibrillation. This arrhythmia is a shivering of the atrial chambers and usually can be dealt without major difficulties. In patients with HOCM, atrial fibrillation should be treated without delay, to avoid quick deterioration of the cardiac function.

WHAT TO DO

- Screening of first-degree relatives by echocardiography is recommended every 3 years for children and young adults and every 5 years thereafter
- Avoid strenuous exercises
- Allow low to moderate levels of aerobic exercises
- Have endocarditis prophylaxis
- The patient should always be well hydrated
- Nitroglycerin or nitrate derivates should be avoided since they can facilitate the obstruction of the left ventricular outflow tract

- Beta-blocker and calcium blockers are valuable
- Those with severe HOCM who do not respond to medical treatment may be considered for heart surgery. One could also undergo septal myectomy, which is a removal of a portion of the thickened septum
- Septal ablation has been successfully tried, and this consists of an injection of 100% alcohol into the first septal perforator artery via cardiac catheterization, purposely causing a myocardial infarction in the thickened septum with atrophy (shrinkage) of the grossly enlarged portion of the heart muscle, and subsequent relief of the obstruction (or most of it). This procedure has its own inherent complications. One of my patients had it done, developed advanced heart block from it, was implanted a permanent pacemaker, and felt "cured." He ran miles every day without any discomfort

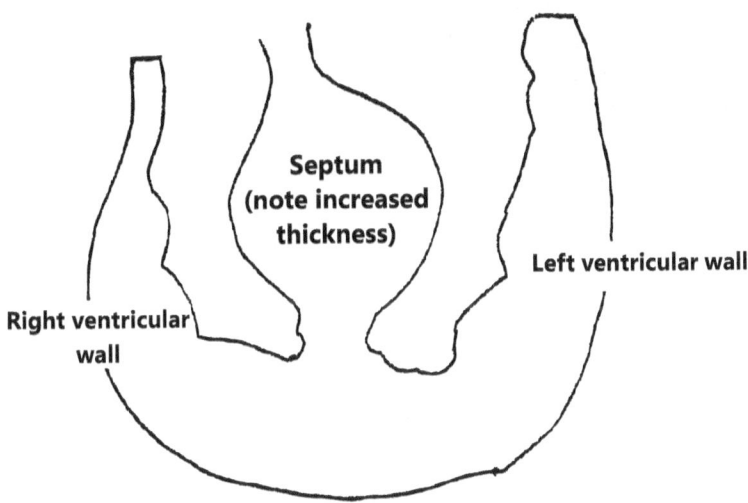

Hypertrophic obstructive cardiomyopathy

Figure 18

RESTRICTIVE, OBLITERATIVE, AND INFILTRATIVE CARDIOMYOPATHIES

These cardiomyopathies occur because different substances infiltrate the heart muscle and its inner layer called the endocardium. They lead to heart failure and arrhythmias not only through involvement of the cardiac muscle but also the conducting or electric system producing all kinds of dangerous arrhythmias and occasionally SCD. The basic dynamic feature of these cardiomyopathies is the stiffness the heart presents to the blood load that returns to its chambers.

89—AMYLOIDOSIS

This consists in deposits of an amyloid protein that infiltrates various organs, the heart included. There are four different types of amyloidosis: one is associated with bone cancer, multiple myeloma; another with chronic infections, such as tuberculosis; a third variety with autoimmnune disease (rheumatoid arthritis); and finally, senile cardiac amyloidosis where the hearts of some elderly people become loaded with amyloid.

This condition may cause heart failure and lethal arrhythmias. In some cases, therapy to neutralize an immunological reaction is used, but the condition does not really have a specific, effective treatment. Serious bradycardias are treated with pacemakers. **Cardiac transplantation should be avoided because the disease invariably comes back and involves the newly transplanted heart.**

90—ENDOMYOCARDIAL FIBROSIS

This disease usually affects children and young adults. The inner layer of the heart, called the endocardium, suffers a process of thickening, causing great stiffness of the heart muscle, and the heart's inability to accommodate the blood it receives. Patients experience shortness of breath, edemas, palpitations, easy fatigability, and have disease of the cardiac valves, arrhythmias, and congestive heart failure. Diagnosis is only firmly established by endomyocardial biopsy. Generally, it is a serious condition although there are milder cases.

91—HEMOCHROMATOSIS

This is an inborn error of metabolism (genes abnormality) that leads to iron deposition in various organs, heart included, and this results in a cardiomyopathy. The acquired variety of hemochromatosis is due to multiple blood transfusions with resulting iron deposits in the heart and other organs, such as the skin, pancreas, liver, the pituitary gland, testicles, and ovaries.

The diagnosis is made when the serum iron and ferritin show elevated blood levels. Final proof is by endomyocardial biopsy. Treatment is repeated phlebotomies (blood extractions). The chelating agent desferrioxamine is useful in binding the iron circulating in the blood. In selected cases, heart transplantation (with or without liver transplantation) may be considered.

For arrhythmogenic right ventricular dysplasia (ARVD), please see section 100.

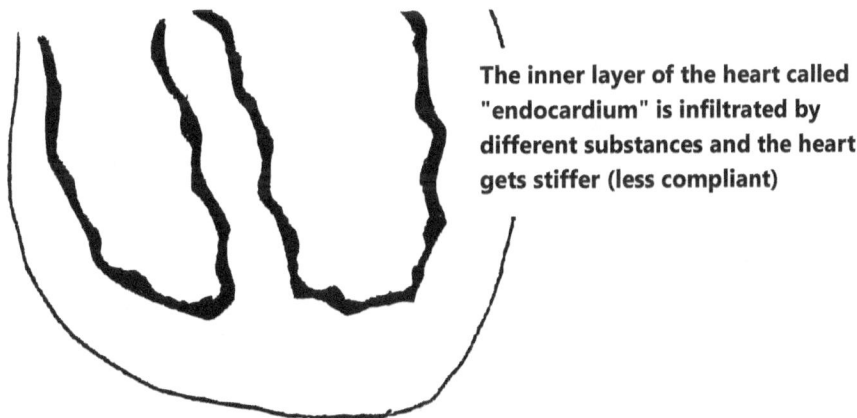

The inner layer of the heart called "endocardium" is infiltrated by different substances and the heart gets stiffer (less compliant)

Restrictive cardiomyopathy

Figure 19

92—NONCOMPACTION CARDIOMYOPATHY

This is a recently described disease (1990). It is an unclassified cardiomyopathy, a genetic disorder that may or may not be associated with other congenital abnormalities. When it is not, it is termed *isolated* noncompaction cardiomyopathy. The theory that attempts to explain this disorder is that there is an intrauterine arrest of myocardial (cardiac muscle) development with lack of compaction of the loose meshwork of ventricular trabeculae. This results in diffuse hypertrophy or enlargement of deep ventricular trabeculations with weakened contractions of different segments of the ventricles. The disease can be identified by echocardiocardiogram, CT scan, and MRI. It may produce no symptoms, or it can cause heart failure and form clots inside the cardiac chambers. These may be released into the general circulation (emboli). Sometimes, life-threatening arrhythmias are present. It's important to implant an intracardiac defibrillation early in the course of the disease to prevent a disastrous arrhythmic event.

DISEASE OF THE HEART VALVES

93—AORTIC STENOSIS

This is a narrowing of the aortic valve orifice that causes an obstruction to the outflow of blood from the left ventricle. The most common causes are congenital, rheumatic, and in elderly individuals, calcific degeneration of the valve. Calcium deposits are as hard as cement, accumulate in the valve leaflets, and little by little reduce the opening of the valve.

Severe aortic stenosis is common in patients 60 years of age or older and lethal if uncorrected, **when the lesion has already produced symptoms** (dizziness, fainting, chest pains and/or shortness of breath, and heart failure). With the onset of severe symptoms (any of the ones just mentioned) the average life expectancy is 2-3 years. Almost all patients with heart failure are deceased in 1-2 years. The survival of patients with severe aortic stenosis is worse than that of many malignancies. **The treatment approach of severe aortic stenosis in the elderly who has *no* symptoms related to that lesion is conservative, which means, no surgery. Close follow-up, however, is indicated since the development of symptoms due to aortic stenosis is an indication to consider aortic valve replacement.**

The incidence of sudden death in AS is estimated to be of about 5%.

The detection of a murmur that proves to be due to aortic stenosis should not be a reason for undue alarm. If the lesion is mild to moderate, it should be followed periodically, usually once a year, to see if it becomes severe. When that happens, aortic valve replacement with a prosthetic valve (mechanical or tissue valve) needs to be considered. Operative mortality is about 4%, and long-term recoveries are common.

All patients with aortic stenosis need antibiotic prophylaxis against infective endocarditis.

Exercise tests should be avoided in patients with severe aortic stenosis. An acceleration of the heart rate imposes a heavy burden on the heart.

The diagnosis is made by physical examination and echocardiography. As a general rule, these are often followed by cardiac catheterization.

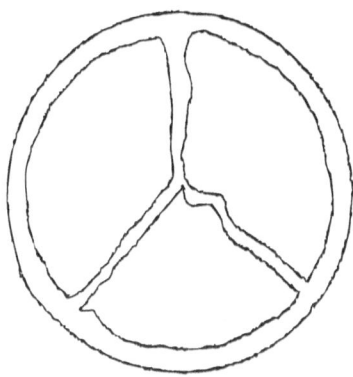

**A—Normal aortic valve
Closed**

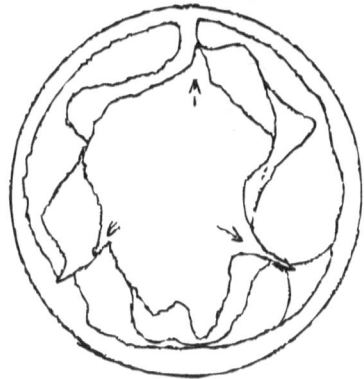

**B—Normal aortic valve
Open**

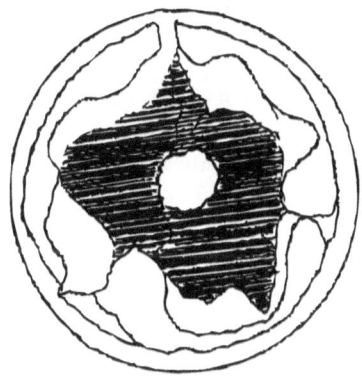

C—Aortic stenosis

The valve in "open" position

Figure 20

94—AORTIC INSUFFICIENCY

This is a leakage of blood that is first ejected by the left ventricle into the circulation, but due to the defective closure of the aortic valve leaflets, a portion of that blood returns to the left ventricle, imposing a burden on it.

When the condition is chronic, it is usually tolerated for a number of years. Its most frequent cause is an arterial wall weakness resulting from degeneration of its medial layer. It could be from rheumatic heart disease, previous episodes of endocarditis, or a congenitally abnormal aortic valve. Normally, the aortic valve has three leaflets (tricuspid). A congenitally abnormal aortic valve has two leaflets (bicuspid).

Patients with chronic mild AR may have a normal life expectancy as long as the lesion does not progress. Sometimes, an episode of endocarditis aggravates the situation by further damaging the valve.

Acute aortic regurgitation is a different story. It presents as an acute event, with severe shortness of breath and acute congestive heart failure, which may be fatal if untreated. Intensive medical therapy is followed as soon as possible by aortic valve replacement.

Surgery may at times wait if the patient's condition stabilizes, but at times, it is required on urgent or emergent basis.

The two most common causes of acute aortic insufficiency or regurgitation (AR) are infection of the aortic valves (infective endocarditis) and prosthetic valve dysfunction. Other causes include severe hypertension, aortic dissection, and trauma.

Disease of the cardiac valves, such as mitral regurgitation (leakage of the mitral valve), aortic stenosis, and aortic regurgitation, if not treated on due time, may progress to left ventricular dilatation and poor left ventricular function.

Severely depressed cardiac function will not improve significantly the left ventricular pumping function after surgical treatment (valve replacement), but still, the patient is better off since the burden of valvular impairment is eliminated.

Valvular lesions are handled differently. For example, severe mitral regurgitation associated with a poor ejection fraction of under 25% poses a prohibited surgical risk. On the other hand, the same ejection fraction in a patient who has severe aortic stenosis gives a green light to proceed with aortic valve replacement.

95—ENDOCARDITIS

This is a life-threatening disease. A few decades ago, the prognosis was dismal. Fortunately, medico-surgical and technological advances have made a big difference.

Rheumatic heart disease (RHD) used to be the most frequent predisposing cause years back. But RHD incidence has decreased, and survivors of congenital heart disease have increased. Illicit drugs, HIV, immunosuppressive therapies, organ transplantation (particularly renal), chronic hemodialysis, diabetes, mitral valve prolapse, and poor dental hygiene are always significant predisposing conditions for infective endocarditis.

Prosthetic valves (mitral or aortic), both biological or mechanic, represent a high risk for IE. In children, congenital cyanotic heart disease such as **Tetralogy of Fallot** is a frequent predisposing abnormality, but others such as **aortic stenosis, ventricular septal defect, pulmonic stenosis, patent ductus arteriosus, and coarctation of the aorta** can be affected too.

Intravenous drug users are 300 times more likely to die with IE than nonusers. They rarely use sterile syringes and needles. Postcardiac surgery patients should always be considered candidates for IE. Pregnancy poses special dangers at the time of delivery, when this complicates with infections of the uterus, septic thrombophlebitis in pelvic veins, or severe urinary tract infections.

Septic abortion or infection associated with an IUD (intrauterine device) may throw profuse number of germs into the bloodstream and cause endocarditis. Hospitalized patients are not exempt: infections caused by surgery and indwelling cathethers, wounds, biopsy sites. The tips (leads) of pacemakers or intracardiac defibrillators catheters inserted in the right ventricle may be the source of a valve infection.

The duration of endocarditis therapy generally varies from 4 to 6 weeks of intravenous antibiotics. After the initial therapy in the hospital, if the course is uncomplicated, treatment may be completed at home. Periodic blood cultures are obtained to verify the success of therapy. Some patients also need to be treated surgically. Some major indications for surgery include moderate or severe heart failure, myocardial abscesses, valvular obstruction, and persistent bacteremia despite appropriate antibiotics.

IE is virtually always fatal if left untreated. A sudden or very rapid death in endocarditis may result from an occlusion of a coronary artery by a vegetation (typical lesion of endocarditis) of the aortic valve, intractable congestive heart failure resulting from the perforation or destruction of a valve leaflet, or rupture of a chordae tendinea. Shock due to septicemia may follow a tragically speedy evolution too.

96—PROSTHETIC HEART VALVE DYSFUNCTION

There are two types of prosthetic heart valves (PHV): mechanical prosthesis with rigid occluders, and biological or tissue valves, with flexible leaflets of human or animal origin (porcine or bovine).

Mechanical valves are the following:

* *Ball valves.* The one type that endured until today is the Starr-Edwards valve
* *Disk valves.* The Bjork-Shiley valve was introduced in 1969. One model, CC (Convexo-Concave) was found to have a structural failure caused by strut fracture I've seen patients many years after implantation, and the valves were working very well.
* *Bileaflet valves.* The St. Jude valve was introduced in 1977. The occluders are two semicircular leaflets

Biological valves include the following:

* *Autograft.* One patient's own valve is translocated (the patient's pulmonary valve is placed in the aortic position)
* *Homograft* (or allograft). A valve is transplanted from another human
* *Heterograft* (or xenograft). A valve is transplanted from another specie (porcine aortic valve or bovine pericardial valve)

The advantage of a mechanical valve is its durability.

The advantage of a tissue valve is that no long term anticoagulation is needed. Its disadvantage is structural valvular deterioration.

There are many potential complications of PHV (prosthethic heart valves). Some of them are serious and can be lethal: endocarditis, major internal or external bleeding associated with the use of anticoagulants, valve thrombosis (occlusion of the valve, aortic or mitral), embolism (a clot from the valve area thrown to the brain). A post-operative complication of valve replacement that needs immediate detection—and attention—is cardiac tamponade due to blood accumulation in the pericardial cavity. This tends to occur during the first 45 days following valve replacement. That pericardial blood needs to be removed **fast**!

I once witnessed in the ICU the sudden death of a man whose doctors had troubles to control his severe hypertension that followed his aortic valve replacement with a ball valve prosthesis. The ball went through the struts, and he was left with nothing to close the valve area. He died in seconds with massive pulmonary edema due to aortic regurgitation. The postmortem examination found the ball in the groin, at the level of the bifurcation of the iliac arteries.

Prosthetic dehiscence is the result of suture failure. Stitches are pulled out of the cardiac tissues. This results from infection, operative technical error, or diseased cardiac tissues (fragile, swollen, calcified).

Sometimes, death occurs in patients who had a normally functioning prosthetic valve, and the cause of the demise is never found.

The echocardiogram (thoracic or/and esophageal) is extremely useful in detecting prosthetic valvular dysfunctions.

All patients with prosthetic valves must have appropriate antibiotics for prophylaxis against endocarditis. Those who required anticoagulation should have it carefully done and have blood tests to assure the proper levels of anticoagulation.

The 4-6 week post-operative visit is critically important and requires a careful physical examination, blood tests, ECG, chest x-ray, echocardiogram, and the INR (international normalized ratio) that measures the degree of anticoagulation.

Some prosthetic valve dysfunctions require a reoperation.

97—DISRUPTION OF THE MITRAL VALVE APPARATUS— SEVERE ACUTE MITRAL REGURGITATION

The mitral valve is located between the left atrium and the left ventricle. It has two leaflets that open and close with each heartbeat. The mitral valve apparatus includes these valves and a support system that keeps the valves' normal function: a mitral ring wrapped around them, the chordae tendinea to which the valve leaflets are attached, and the papillary muscles that connect with the chordae tendinea that are inserted in the ventricle muscular tissue.

Different disorders may affect any of the structures of the mitral valve apparatus. For example, **severe mitral valve prolapse (MVP)** associated with mitral regurgitation may one day turned into an acute emergency. I had a fifty-year-old male patient whom I followed for twenty years and who had severe MVP with good tolerance except for occasional short-lasting palpitations. One night, he developed acute heart failure. **The cause was the rupture of a chordae tendineae.** The mitral valve leaked blood back to the lungs, and these were filled up with fluid. He had successful valve replacement.

MVP and Sudden Death

MVP appears to slightly increase the risk of sudden death in patients with severe mitral regurgitation, complex arrhythmias, and a history of severe palpitations and/or syncope.

Patients who have mild mitral valve prolapse usually have an excellent prognosis and carry out normal physical activities and may have mild symptoms or no symptoms. Prolapsed mitral valves are composed of a loose material with fragmented, disorganized, prominent collagen fibers, and sometimes there is an association with connective tissue disorders.

Infection of the mitral valve (endocarditis) can perforate the valve leaflet and cause acute mitral valve insufficiency and pulmonary edema.

Rupture of a papillary muscle during an acute myocardial infarction causes extremely severe mitral regurgitation and is usually fatal. Surgical treatment aims at reattaching the papillary muscle to the ventricular wall. Mortality with this kind of treatment is high, but it's worse without it. In some cases, if the rupture papillary muscle is not complete and the patient can be stabilized medically, it is preferable to defer the operation for 4-6 weeks after the acute myocardial infarction.

In other cases of severe mitral regurgitation, the mitral valve needs to be either reconstructed or replaced. Surgical mortality depends on the function of the left ventricle and on the presence of coexisting conditions such as renal, liver, or pulmonary disease.

98—CARDIAC TAMPONADE

This is an accumulation of fluid in the pericardial cavity.

The heart is normally surrounded by a membrane called the pericardium that has two layers with a small amount of fluid in between them.

An abnormal accumulation of fluid in the pericardial space may be seen in patients who have no symptoms, and when it is small to moderate, it may be carried for decades without any evidence of disease. The origin of this fluid accumulation at times is never known, and its discovery is incidental.

Perforation of the left ventricular wall due to an acute myocardial infarction may cause a sudden or rapid death due to the flow of blood into the pericardium that produces cardiac tamponade.

The majority of effusions of moderate size or greater that result in cardiac tamponade **are caused by pericardial injury and/or inflammation. Stab and bullet wounds or acute viral pericarditis are usually responsible.**

Pericardial effusions per se are usually symptom free unless they are complicated by cardiac compression.

Actually, the amount of accumulated pericardial fluid does not necessarily determine the patient's deterioration of his or her clinical status. Critical tamponade can occur from as little as 60-100 ml of blood when acutely introduced into the pericardial sac or may require more than one liter of slowly accumulating fluid. In such cases, intrapericardial pressure increases and compresses the heart affecting its function.

When the increased amount of pericardial fluid reaches a crucial level, the cardiac output (the amount of blood ejected by the heart into the general circulation per minute) is reduced, and cardiovascular collapse ensues.

Accumulating pericardial fluid causes a rapid pulse and dyspnea (shortness of breath), poor appetite (anorexia), profound weakness, cold clammy extremities, restlessness, and mental confusion and stupor.

The presence of abnormal amount of pericardial fluid can be easily detected by cardiac ultrasound (echocardiography). Drainage of this fluid is the only effective treatment and should be done on urgent or emergent basis, depending upon individual circumstances. Echocardiographically guided transcutaneous (through the skin) pericardiocentesis (a needle introduced into the pericardial cavity) is quite a safe procedure. Sometimes, a pericardiotomy (a small incision under the sternal bone) creates a "window" in the pericardium and evacuates the fluid effectively too.

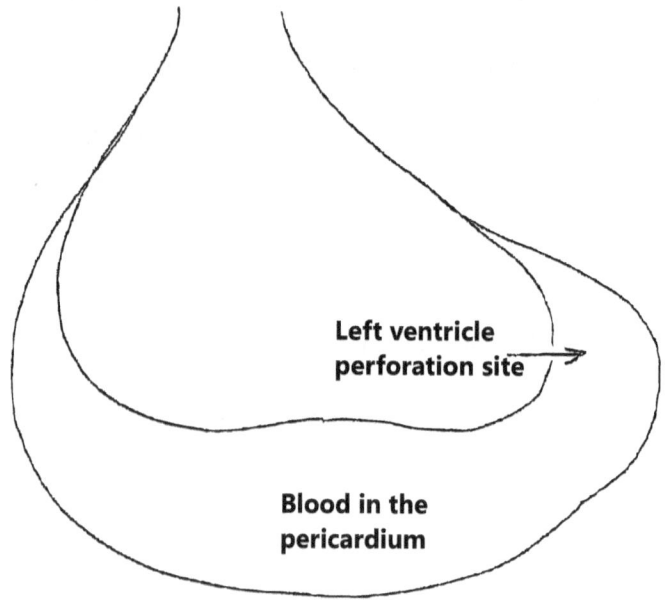

Left ventricle perforation site

Blood in the pericardium

Pericardial tamponade due to rupture of the left ventricular wall (acute myocardial infarction)

Figure 21

99—TRAUMATIC INJURIES TO THE HEART

The first time a heart wound was sutured in the United States was by Dr. Hill in 1902, on a kitchen table. Injuries to the heart may be penetrating or blunt.

In the United States, trauma is the fourth leading cause of death and the leading cause of death in those younger than forty years of age. Traumas to the heart are classified according to the mechanism of the provoking injury

- **Penetrating**
  Gunshot wounds: handgun, rifle, other projectiles
  Stab sounds: knives, ice picks, swords, fence posts, wire

- **Nonpenetrating (blunt)**
  Motor vehicle (seat belt, air bag)
  Crushing
  Falls from height
  Blasts (explosives, grenades)
  Fracture of sternum
  Fracture ribs
  Sports, e.g., baseball

- **Medically induced (iatrogenic)**
  Cardiac catheters
  Fluid extraction from the pericardium by needle aspiration

- **Others**
  Electrical
  Burn (*)
  Missile entering a vein or an artery that travels to the heart (embolization)

(*) *I recently saw a woman in her twenties who was found to have an abnormal ECG and echocardiogram-Doppler study. The latter shows mild impairment of the left ventricular function and moderate regurgitation of her tricuspid valve. The origin of these abnormalities was uncertain. However, when she was five years of age, she had a third-degree burn in her anterior chest and had been in coma for five days. It is highly probable that her heart was damaged by the intense heat of her thoracic burn.*

The most frequent **penetrating injury** to the heart observed in hospitals is due to stab wounds. Sixty to one hundred milliliter of blood acutely entering the pericardial cavity may compress the heart and impair its functioning (cardiac tamponade). Injuries to the right atrium and right ventricle and coronary arteries can be very serious, but an injury to the left ventricle may lead to cardiac arrest in seconds.

Penetrating heart trauma is highly lethal, and most patients don't reach the hospital alive. This is the most frequently seen cardiac injury in hospitals. Some mechanisms include gunshot wounds, stab wounds, ice picks, fence impalements. Due to their anatomic position, the right and left ventricles are at greater risk than the atrial chambers. Although some cardiac injuries present with a cardiac arrest, no pulse, no blood pressure, no respiration, others show the patient alert, comfortable, and with normal vital signs. But not for too long: up to 80% of stab wounds ultimately produce pericardial tamponade.

Nonpenetrating or blunt cardiac injury can be caused by compression of the heart between the sternum and the vertebral column, e.g., external cardiac massage done during cardiopulmonary resuscitation (CPR).

Other blunt injuries may result from falls, vehicular accidents, and blasts. A baseball hitting the chest at an electrically vulnerable period of the cardiac cycle may end a person's life. (See "Commotion Cordis" at section 125.)

Medically induced injuries, also called iatrogenic, can occur even when procedures are performed by highly trained and skillful operators. Catheters may perforate a coronary artery or the heart muscle or dissect the aorta. When these threaten a catastrophic outcome, an emergent operation must be done.

The incidence of coronary artery perforation with balloon angioplasty is estimated to be 0.1-0.2%, but with more complex and advanced procedures such as coronary artery stenting, atherectomy, rotablation or laser ablation, the incidence may be as high as 3%.

For electricity-caused deaths, please see section titled "Electrocution."

Burns

Cardiac complications of severe body burns may be deadly in the early postburn period. There may be a tear of valve leaflets, rupture of papillary muscle or chordae tendinea, any or all of the above resulting in severe heart failure and a dysfunctional cardiac muscle. Arrhythmias may degenerate into ventricular fibrillation.

TREATMENT

Most individuals with significant cardiac injury don't reach the hospital alive. They have the best chances when they are directly transported (if at all possible) to a trauma center. Chances for survival improve when the patient is immediately introduced an endotracheal tube to assist the respiratory function and transport time is less than five minutes. In these emergencies, every second counts. In the hospital, the heart's surgical exposure is carried out, and multiple abnormalities need intense and concentrated attention, e.g., relief of tamponade, acidosis (accumulation of toxic acids in the blood), hypothermia (very low body temperature), respiratory support, blood transfusions, and much more.

The treatment approach to these patients requires excellent professionals working as a team. Placing stitches in a heart wound (cardiorrhaphy) requires an experience surgeon. Improper technique may damage the coronary arteries or cause enlargement of the laceration under treatment. Sometimes, it is preferable to apply pressure to the wound with a finger and wait for a more experience surgeon.

Trauma centers are intense, impressive, dramatic, high-voltage places. Most people don't realize the drama that is constantly lived in these units, the dedication, and the long hours that health care professionals invest trying to save the lives of persons who often look more dead than alive, and often with mutilated and terribly damaged bodies. The cardiac wound may be severe enough to kill the victim, but quite often, there are so many other wounds that it's difficult to find a tiny healthy spot in the patient's body.

ARRHYTHMIAS: WHEN THE CARDIAC RHYTHM GOES CRAZY . . . AND DANGEROUS!

The heartbeat results from the contraction of the heart. The left ventricle acts as a pump that ejects blood into the circulatory system. The pulse taken from any artery of the body represents the blood that was sent to that artery by the contraction of the left ventricle. What I just described is a mechanical action of the heart. But what gives the heart muscle the power to contract? The answer is an electrical current that originates in a tiny battery—like structure called the sinus node (SN), located at the right atrium, and is transmitted to the rest of the heart by a series of bundles that form the **electrical or conducting system of the heart.**

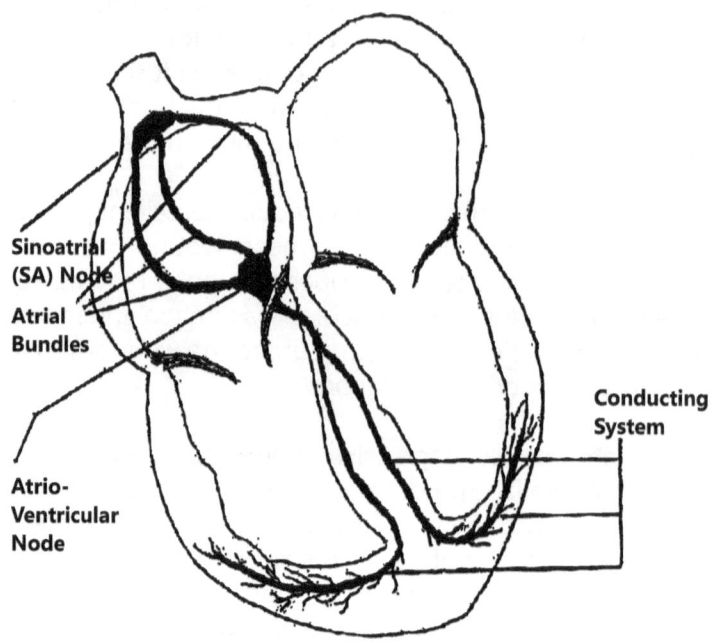

Sinoatrial
(SA) Node

Atrial
Bundles

Conducting
System

Atrio-
Ventricular
Node

Conducting system of the heart

Figure 22

The heart's electrical activity originates in an area located in the right atrium called the sinus node (SN). This tiny but extremely important structure measures 1-2 cm long and 0.5 cm wide. It is called the natural pacemaker of the heart. From here, the generated electrical current spreads through several bundles to the atrial chambers, and they converge to reach the atrioventricular node (AVN). As the current keeps on descending, it reaches the interventricular septum, the portion of heart tissue that separates both ventricles. The interventricular septum has two bundles: the right and the left. The electrical wave travels through both of them and reach the so-called His-Purkinje conduction system, which spreads the current to the rest of the heart muscle. Electrical energy is converted to mechanical energy, and the heart contracts.

The ECG (electrocardiogram), at times called the EKG (from German *electrokardiogram*), records the electrical activity of the heart as much as the electroencephalogram registers the electrical activity of the brain. The ECG was discovered a century ago. That electrical activity is detected by electrodes applied to your extremities (arms and legs) and the left side of the anterior chest. What the ECG registers are "waves" that form a graph. The electrodes' function is to pick up the heart's electrical activity from different angles.

The main components of an ECG reading are the P waves, the QRS complex, and the T wave. Each ECG complex represents a heartbeat.

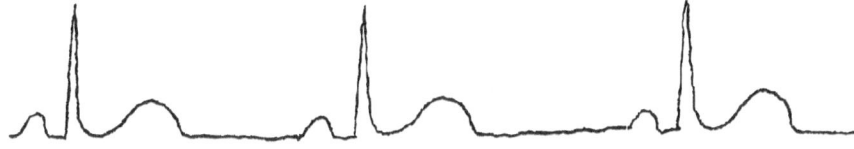

Normal cardiac rhythm

Figure 23

The P wave represents the passing of electrical activity through the atria.

Following the P wave is the PR interval, a flat section that represents the time the impulse travels through the atrioventricular node (AVN).

The QRS complex occurs as the electrical wave travels through the ventricles.

The T wave is formed during the time the heart muscle recovers electrically and gets ready for the next beat.

The ECG is the best way to diagnose any cardiac rhythm abnormality. The normal rhythm is called sinus rhythm. There are multiple rhythm abnormalities. We are not going to discuss them in this book.

Disturbances in the conducting system produce reactions of different kinds and severity. Abnormalities of the conducting system may cause slowing of the heart rate (bradycardia), acceleration of the heartbeat (tachycardia), and an abundant number of irregularities. Some of these are trivial and extremely common and have no pathological meaning. Others are significant because they can induce palpitations, shortness of breath, chest pains, dizziness or fainting. Sometimes, arrhythmias can be dangerous and deadly. Please see cardiac arrest, VT, VF, asystole, and sick sinus syndrome (section 40 and 104).

100—ARRHYTHMOGENIC RIGHT VENTRICULAR DYSPLASIA (ARVD)

This is an infrequent cause of sudden death. It is more common in some parts of the world, and there's a familial incidence of this disorder in about 30% of cases. It is a form of cardiomyopathy that predominantly (not exclusively) involves the right ventricle. The walls of the right ventricle become very thin, and fatty tissue replaces the normal myocardium. Its prevalence is 1 per 5,000 but in northern Italy is more frequent (4.4 per 1,000).

In the United States it accounts for about 5% of unexplained sudden deaths in the young and up to 20% in Italy.

This disease typically shows a young man (there's a male predominance) with frequent ventricular premature beats, but at times sudden death is the initial (and final) manifestation.

Ventricular tachycardia (VT) is the characteristic arrhythmia of this condition and is often precipitated by exercise. VT has a characteristic ECG pattern. Electrophysiological study is necessary. A definite diagnosis of ARVD is achieved when a microscopic examination of right ventricular muscle (during surgery o biopsy) shows its replacement by fatty tissue.

CMR or cardiac magnetic resonance is by far the most sensitive noninvasive method for the diagnosis. MRI findings that suggest ARVD include dilatation of both the right atrium and right ventricle and an aneurysm at the tip (apex) of the right ventricle.

The outlook of patients who suffer from this disease is unpredictable. Vigorous physical activities are not advisable due to the known tendency of these patients to develop malignant arrhythmias during exertions. Some patients with nonlife threatening arrhythmias are considered for treatment with drugs or ablation. However, when the disorder has a familial incidence, syncope (loss of consciousness), evidence of right ventricular disease, and life-threatening rhythm disturbances, an ICD implantation is indicated.

101—BRUGADA SYNDROME: SLEEP DEATH IN JAPAN AND SOUTHEAST ASIA

This disorder is characterized by sporadic runs of ventricular tachycardia, ventricular fibrillation, a family history of sudden death in members younger than forty-five years of age, nocturnal and agonal respiration, and for those who are familiar with electrocardiography, the ECG characteristically shows a right bundle branch block with persistent ST segment elevation in V1 and V2 in patients without structural heart disease.

A similar syndrome has been described in young, apparently healthy males from Southeast Asia, and the disease is described with different names in different countries. The Thai call it *lai tai* (death during the sleep). In the Philippines, it is known as *bangungut* (moan in sleep followed by death).

The Japanese named it *pokkuri* (unexpected sudden death at night). This condition is genetically determined, and most of the affected are of Asian origin.

Patients who have this disorder and experience palpitations and tachycardias have a high incidence of SCD (sudden cardiac death). There is a lower incidence of SCD in those who show the ECG abnormalities but never had any symptoms and do not have inducible ventricular tachycardia on electrophysiological testing. Most experts agree that implantation of an ICD in this group of patients does not provide benefit. Patients with Brugada who have syncope, VT (ventricular tachycardia), or a cardiac arrest should be treated with an ICD.

102—ELECTROLYTE IMBALANCE

Hypokalemia (low blood levels of potassium) may cause life-threatening arrhythmias, particularly in those suffering from an acute myocardial infarction or those who are taking digitalis with a diuretic that eliminated through the urine substantial amounts of potassium through the urine.

Other common causes of severe hypokalemia are severe eating disorders (anorexia, bulimia) and protein liquid diets. Magnesium deficiency (e.g., alcoholism) may also cause a cardiac arrest.

103—SLOW HEART RATES: CARDIAC STANDSTILL, SICK SINUS SYNDROME (SSS), ADVANCED HEART BLOCK, HYPERSENSITIVE CAROTID SINUS

The normal heart rates vary from 60 to 100 beats per minute. Bradycardia means a slow heart rate. Heart rates between 20 and 40 beats per minute usually cause a fainting spell. The cause of such bradycardia is a sick sinus syndrome (SSS) or advanced heart block (AHB). At times, the heart stops altogether, and all the ECG shows is a straight line. Unless it is reversed and a functional heart rhythm resumes, the outcome is fatal.

SSS results from dysfunction of the sinus node. When disease affects it (aging, atherosclerotic heart disease, cardiomyopathy, drugs), the little battery runs out of charge and becomes sluggish.

Advanced heart block means that the sinus node is working well, but the conducting system of the heart below it is unable to transmit the electrical current to the ventricles. As a desperate reaction, the ventricle creates its own beats, but does it at a very slow rate and that leads to fainting, heart failure, or more chest pains.

The treatment for both of the above is the implantation of a permanent pacemaker.

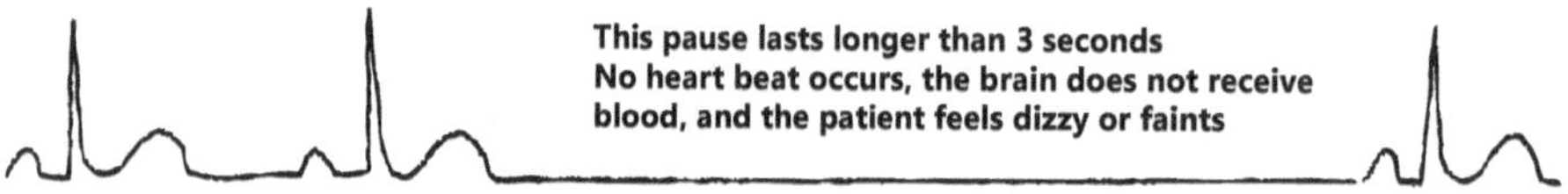

This pause lasts longer than 3 seconds
No heart beat occurs, the brain does not receive blood, and the patient feels dizzy or faints

Sick Sinus Syndrome (SSS)

Figure 24

104—IDIOPATHIC VENTRICULAR TACHYCARDIA (VT) AND VENTRICULAR FIBRILLATION (VF)

The term *idiopathic* means that the origin of a disturbance is unknown. In the last few years, great advances were made in the understanding of cases of SCD produced by VF sometimes preceded by VT. We described some of them, such as the **catecholaminergic VT,** caused by a significant increase in the blood-circulating catecholamines, a short or prolonged QT interval, cocaine-induced VT and VF, among others. But still there are some individuals who develop cardiac arrest, and no structural heart disease can be identified. These cases are called idiopathic ventricular fibrillation. This disorder is higher in selected populations such as children or patients younger than 40 years of age.

Anyone who survives a cardiac arrest due to spontaneous VF should always be evaluated by a cardiologist who specializes in electrophysiology. The latest technological developments offer plenty of hope to prevent or treat this condition.

105—PROLONGED QT INTERVAL—THE LONG QT SYNDROME

The QT interval represents a portion of the electrical complex that produces each heartbeat.

Patients who have a prolonged QT have a propensity to develop malignant ventricular arrhythmias and sudden death, particularly associated with extreme emotional reactions and strenuous physical exertions.

Some patients with hereditary prolonged QT intervals suffer from deafness while others do not. Syncopal episodes (total loss of consciousness) are a frequent expression of this disease. Treatment includes beta-blockers, pacemaker or ICD implantation.

Acquired Long QT Syndrome

There are numerous causes for this abnormality including the following:

* *Number of antiarrhythmic drugs.* Some of them are quinidine, procainamide, disopyramide, sotalol, amiodarone
* *Noncardiac drugs.* Examples are the following: Haldol, antihistamines (terfenadine, astemizole), antibiotics (e.g., erythromycin, sulfamethoxazole/trimethoprim), chemotherapeutic agents (e.g., pentamidine, anthracycline)
* *Nutritional deficiencies.* These are deficiencies associated with unregulated weight-reducing diets such as hypocalcemia, hypothyroidism, intracranial hemorrhage, hypokalemia, and hypomagnesemia.

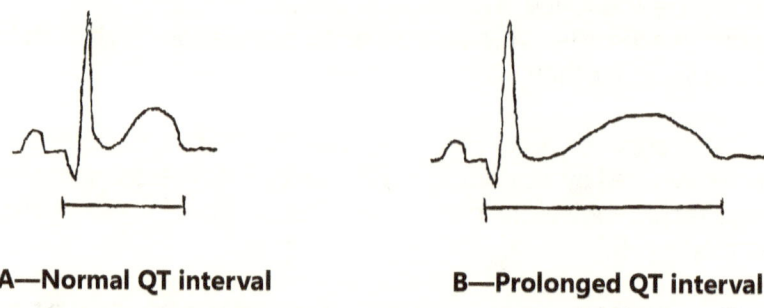

A—Normal QT interval   **B—Prolonged QT interval**

Figure 25

106—SHORT QT INTERVAL SYNDROME

This is a recently recognized entity (it was described for the first time in year 2000). It is capable of leading to lethal arrhythmias. Patients may experience palpitations and/or syncope. Some drugs such as sotalol and ibutilide have been used to prolong the QT, but the implantation of an intracardiac defibrillator should be seriously considered.

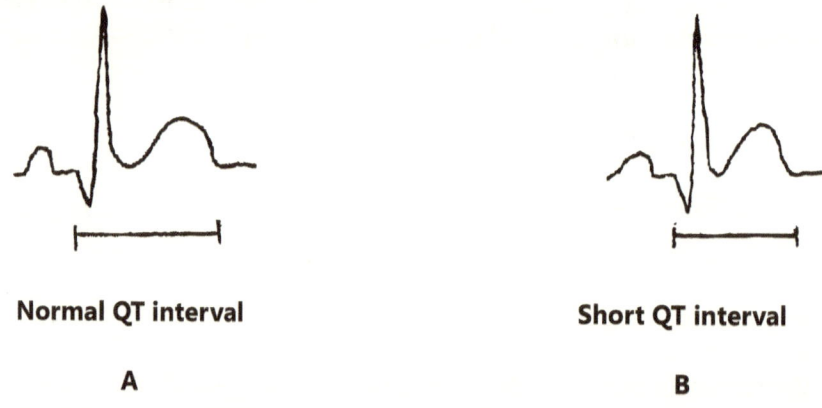

Normal QT interval   **Short QT interval**

A   **B**

Figure 26

107—PACEMAKER FAILURE

Pacemakers are lifesaving devices. There are different types. Some of them are implanted because the patient's heart rate falls to unacceptable levels, usually causing fainting spells. Some units are useful to manage heart failure.

No mechanical device is exempt from potential failures. I'll mention some of them:

- *Runaway pacemaker.* This is an uncommon and yet potentially lethal circuit malfunction that produces an erratic, very rapid rhythm. **The approach is to deactivate and the pacemaker immediately**
- *Lead failure.* The pacemaker leads are placed in various cardiac chambers depending upon the characteristics of the arrhythmias being treated. These leads may suffer long-term complications. One of them is a **current leak** and failure to deliver the pacing signal to the heart muscle. The malfunction may be intermittent and not detectable by a routine examination
- *Failure to capture.* Leads may also fracture and fail to pace the heart. When that happens, the outcome depends upon the patient's own rhythm. If it is slow but functional, the heart continues to beat although the patient may feel exhausted, dizzy, or faint. A potentially lethal situation happens if the pacemaker fails to act, and the patient has a prolonged period of time without any heartbeat
- *Failure to output.* The pacemaker may suffer from absence of pacing stimuli. This means no capture. Capture of the cardiac muscle by the pacemaker means that the pacemaker electrical stimuli is delivered effectively and allows the contraction of the heart
- *Oversensing and undersensing.* Sensing is the capacity of the pacemaker system to react to signals resulting from the patient's own heartbeat. The dysfunction may go both ways: too much sensing or too little sensing. Both abnormalities may lead to rhythm disturbances, but specialists in this highly technological field find ways to fix the dysfunction
- *Electromagnetic interference (EMI):* This results from an electrical signal (outside the patient's own body) that interferes with pacemaker function. Various sources inside a hospital or outside may cause problems

In the hospital environment, the most common sources of EMI include electrocautery and defibrillation. These can stop the pacemaker functioning, and if the patient is pacemaker dependent (this means that without the pacemaker help the patient does not have a viable cardiac rhythm), the heart rate may become very slow (bradycardia) or non-existent (asystole). Cautery should be avoided near a pacemaker.

As far as defibrillation, the pads should be applied in the anteroposterior position (one in the front, left side, and the other

in the back) rather than the anteroapical position, which is one pad in the left side of the chest around the nipple area and another pad below it.

Both electrocautery and defibrillation may damage the pacemaker permanently.

Other sources of EMI in the hospital include lithotripsy, MRI, diathermy, radiofrequency, catheter ablation, transcutaneous electric nerve stimulator (TENS), and spinal cord stimulators.

Additional sources of EMI include digital cellular phones, electronic article surveillance devices, metal detectors, electric razors, high-voltage power lines, welding, transformers, and electric motors.

Digital cell phones should not be placed in the pocket on the side where the pacemaker is located. Electronic surveillance devices or antitheft devices currently used in stores and libraries can cause transient pacemaker malfunction. So if you have a pacemaker and need to go through any of these places, do it fast.

The following electrical devices do not produce interference: electric can openers, electric shavers, stereos, television, microwave ovens, and electric lawnmowers.

108—WOLF-PARKINSON-WHITE SYNDROME WITH RAPID ATRIAL FIBRILLATION

The heart's electrical cables are plugged the wrong way!

The WPW syndrome (Wolf-Parkinson-White Syndrome) became known in 1920 when these authors published a paper reporting eleven cases. It probably doesn't mean anything to you, and it is possible you never heard of it unless you were diagnosed this condition, have a relative who has it, or you are a health care practitioner familiar with medical terms. It is recognized by its typical ECG features.

This is an unusual and yet very important cardiac disorder. Many patients have an electrocardiogram showing the abnormality and never have any symptoms. Others have intermittent palpitations, and in rare cases, the WPW syndrome may cause a sudden death.

I followed a patient who suffered from palpitations for many years and had serious arrhythmias due to WPW. One day I had a conversation with her that made history (at least, for me!).

What really occurred that day is unusual and weird. I'll relate the story to you in a few moments. I'll do it after telling you a bit more about this disturbance.

HOW THE HEART GENERATES AND TRANSMITS ELECTRICAL SIGNALS

Normally, the heart produces and conducts electricity. The first electrical charge is generated in a tiny area located at the right atrium (sinus node). The electrical current spreads to both upper cardiac chambers (atria) and then to the lower chambers (ventricles). One tiny little "bridge" exists between the atria and the ventricles called the atrioventricular node (AVN).

Some people are born with one or more accessory bundles. These are connections between the atria and the ventricles that "bypass" the AVN. The abnormalities may cause tachycardias. Since the ventricles get the electrical wave earlier than when it is transmitted throughout the AVN, the condition is also known as preexcitation.

The WPW anomaly is a typical, recognizable pattern in the electrocardiogram.

The WPW affects 0.15-0.25% of the general population. The incidence of sudden death ranges from 0.15-0.39%.

It is very unusual to have a cardiac arrest as the initial manifestation of WPW.

Commonly, the patient previously complained of palpitations, dizziness, or fainting. WPW tachycardias have different severity. The most feared and dangerous arrhythmia in patients with WPW is rapid atrial fibrillation. Here, the heart rates are so fast, sometimes around 300 per minute, that the heart has no time to fill the coronary arteries properly. As a result, the myocardium doesn't get enough oxygen and, if uncorrected, quickly ends in ventricular fibrillation and death.

HOW IS WPW TREATED

Patients without any symptoms usually don't need treatment. Catheter ablation is currently considered first-line therapy and the treatment of choice for patients with WPW syndrome. It is curative in more than 95% of patients and with low incidence of complications.

Ablation eliminates the accessory bypass. This is done with radiofrequency catheter ablation. Here, a flexible tube called a catheter is advanced to the heart, and the place of the abnormality is located and dealt with. When successful, the tachycardias disappear, and there is no need for drug therapy.

The treatment of WPW then varies from patient to patient. Some patients need no treatment, just observation and follow-up. Others need highly specialized treatment best provided by a cardiologist who specializes in electrophysiology.

With the available newest technologies involving drugs and ablation, patients with WPW can be treated safely and effectively.

And now, a personal story about one of my patients who suffered from WPW syndrome.

Rose was seventy-two and had been my patient for twenty years. She suffered from severe WPW tachycardias, which we controlled with medications. Ablation was not available then.

One day, during an office visit, she was sad and depressed because her granddaughter had been diagnosed with leukemia. I felt bad about the news and shared her feelings. Up until this point, everything in our encounter was rational and made sense. What followed didn't!

Since I was a child I had an extremely sensitive skin and couldn't tolerate any kind of wool or other irritating clothes. So much so that on occasions, I avoided underwear because the elastic bands to hold them bothered me very much.

The day I had this conversation with Rose, I had no underwear.

While Rose was telling me how devastated she was about her granddaughter's cancer, I realized that my long white coat was unbuttoned, and my pants' zipper was down.

Imagine! My zipper down, and I had no underwear!

So I reacted instinctively and brusquely pulled up the zipper, but I did it so fast that in the process I trapped my genital hair with the zipper. The resulting pain was the most intense I've ever had.

Rose was unaware of my physical pain and kept on crying her misfortune. To act compassionately, I kept on looking at her eyes, but my trapped hair was causing so much pain that I started pouring tears.

Rose mistakenly thought that my tears were coming from her conversation and told me:

"I'm so sorry, Dr. Chapunoff. It wasn't my intention to make you feel so sad!"

PART 6

OTHER CAUSES OF SUDDEN OR RAPID DEATH

109—ABDOMINAL TRAUMA

I was working at the emergency department of a major city hospital when a man in his forties pushed the door of the examining room and asked for help. He had been involved in a fight against another individual. Both of them used knives. He had an open abdominal wound and was holding his intestines with his bare hands. He was relaxed, drunk, humorous, and standing on his feet. A minute later, another man, the one who had stabbed his abdomen, walked in with a deep knife wound that displayed an interesting itinerary. It went from the scalp down the forehead, cut the nose in half, and the palate in half. He was also heavily intoxicated with alcohol and was laughing out loud. Both of them recovered.

TYPES OF ABDOMINAL TRAUMA

1—Penetrating Trauma
* Shotgun wounds (SGW)
* Gunshot wound (GSW)
* Stabbing (SW)

2—Nonpenetrating Trauma
* Compression
* Crush
* Seat belt
* Acceleration/deceleration

Penetrating Trauma

The handgun has replaced the knife as the most common cause of penetrating trauma. It is important to remember that a wound in the upper abdomen may have extended to the thoracic cavity, and a penetrating injury to the chest inferior to the nipples or the tip of the scapula is more likely to cause an intra-abdominal than an intrathoracic injury. If the patient is in shock, probably an important vein or artery has been disrupted.

Gunshot wounds may have a circuitous trajectory involving multiple organs. Knife abdominal wounds may cause bleeding, shock, or peritoneal irritation. **All penetrating abdominal wounds need surgical exploration.**

The liver is the organ more frequently involved (37%) followed by the small bowel (26 %); the stomach, 19%; the colon, 14%; spleen, 7%; kidney, pancreas, duodenum, diaphragm 3-5% each.

Nonpenetrating Trauma

Blunt trauma may be very difficult to evaluate, particularly if the patient is unconscious. The surgeon must decide when to intervene with an abdominal exploratory procedure. In blunt abdominal injuries, the spleen is involved 26% of the times, the kidney 24%, small bowel 16%, liver 15%, pancreas, mesentery, abdominal wall, and diaphragm 1-3% each.

The treatment of both penetrating and nonpenetrating abdominal injuries requires a knowledgeable and experienced surgeon. Lots of attention must be paid to every detail preoperatively, intraoperatively, and post-operatively. In addition, the airways, the heart and circulatory system, and infections deserve special attention.

110—ACCIDENTS

WHAT ARE THE ODDS OF BEING KILLED?

Prevention is the best treatment.

The information that follows is based on the **National Safety Council**'s odds of dying statistics.

The table has four columns. The first column describes the manner of injury (fall, fire, vehicle crash, etc.). The second column gives the total number of deaths in the United States due to the mentioned injuries in 2003. The third column gives the odds of dying in one year due to the manner of injury. The fourth column shows the lifetime odds or chances of dying with the listed injuries.

The original table is far more extensive than the sample shown below.

For more complete information, see data by the National Safety Council **(NSC)**. *National Geographic* magazine's August 2006 issue features the "Ways to Go" chart based on the NSC.

Odds of Death due to Injury, United States, 2003.

Type of Accident	Deaths	One-Year Odds	Lifetime Odds
All external causes of mortality	166,857	1,743	22
Motor vehicle accidents	44,757	6,498	84
Pedestrian	5,991	48,548	626
Motorcycle rider	3,676	79,121	1,020
Car occupant	15,797	18,412	237
Drowning	412	705,947	9,097
Air transport accidents	742	391,981	5,051
Fall on or from stairs and steps	1,588	183,155	2,360
Firearms discharge	730	398,425	5,134
Accidental suffocation and strangulation in bed	497	585,211	7,541
Inhalation of food causing obstruction of the respiratory tract	875	322,400	4,284
Electric transmission lines	96	3,029,688	39,042
Exposure to smoke, fire, and flames	3,369	86,331	1,113

Accidents are the third leading cause of death for males in the United States and the seventh cause of death in women.

TYPES OF ACCIDENTAL DEATHS, USA

2002

	PERCENT
1—Motor vehicle	44.3%
2—Falls	17.8%
3—Poison	13.0%
4—Drowning	3.9%
5—Fires, burns, smoke	3.4%
6—Medical/surgical complications	3.1%
7—Other land transport	1.5%
8—Firearms	0.8%
9—Other (nontransport)	17.8%

Buses are safer: per passenger mile, an **automobile** is 25 times more likely to lead to death than a bus.

Driving under the influence of alcohol is the most important cause of death in car accidents. The second most important is fatigue.

Alcohol below the intoxication levels is also dangerous because it impairs judgment and physical function.

Interestingly, **more than a third of pedestrians killed by a motor vehicle in 1992 were intoxicated.**

The odds of being killed during a scheduled **airline flight** are about one per million, nearly four times greater than the odds of being killed in an automobile ride. But most car trips involve fewer miles. Per passenger mile, an automobile ride is 10 times more likely to result in fatality than an airplane journey.

Most of the **airplanes** fatalities take place during takeoff and landing, mostly the former. The majority of **boating** deaths are due to drowning—with 80% of those dying not wearing life jackets.

Forty percent of **fire** victims die in their sleep.

The death rate per driven mile is **more than 35 times higher for motorcycles than it is for cars.**

The biggest cause of motorcycle accident deaths is car-driver negligence. Vehicle drivers do not pay attention and ignore the presence of motorcyclists on the road.

Hospitals accidents can be dangerous too: many people die annually due to hospital-acquired infections.

CAR ACCIDENT PREVENTION

- Your seatbelt must be buckled
- Pay attention to the road
- Child safety seats must be used correctly
- Drive defensively
- Be always awake and alert
- Don't drink before or while driving. Any amount of alcohol impairs your ability to drive safely
- If you're drunk, don't drive at all: you could kill yourself and/or kill or maim others.
- Avoid excessive speed
- Avoid being distracted
- Don't trust any driver on the road. Many of those who drive suffer from various mental illnesses, dementia, very poor vision, severe hearing impairment, recurrent fainting spells, or vertigo attacks. Some are immature and irresponsible or stressed out. Once in a while, an accident is caused because the driver was engaged in oral-genital sex while driving
- Check traffic before pulling out
- Make sure you respect the Stop or Yield signs and also that **others** coming in the opposite direction do the same. Always check for oncoming vehicles
- Avoid passing without checking traffic **first**

THE WRONG PEOPLE ON THE ROAD

I once had an elderly patient who suffered from advanced dementia. His wife told me that for "the last five years he barely said one word." One day, he spread his feces with his fingers on the living room walls. His upset wife asked him:

"Abe, why did you spread your shit on the wall? Why did you do such a thing? Did you try to tell me something? If so, tell me what it is."

This was his reply: "That's life!"

*She was very proud of him because for the first time in years he pronounced three words. And then she told me: "Dr. Chapunoff, **would you believe that my husband drives me every day to places? He does it very, very well.**"*

I told her: "You're going to sign a paper right now stating that your husband will never drive again. Your husband is a public danger and so are you for allowing him to drive. If he does it again, I'll report you to the police."

And then, you wonder why some freak accidents occur every day.

MOTORCYCLE ACCIDENT PREVENTION

- A helmet is essential. Full face helmets offer better protection
- Helmeted riders are less likely to sustain neck injuries
- Attend a riding school
- Regular practice of hard braking techniques (this means the front brake and the back brakes together)
- Suitable protective gear makes a big difference
- Wear bright, solid, colored riding gear: it avoids accidents
- Experience in driving a motorcycle matters a great deal
- Excess speed is an invitation for trouble
- Any amount of alcohol welcomes tragedy
- A cold rider is as dangerous as a drunk driver
- Surface hazards, e.g., gravel, oil, is a major cause of accidents
- Your best bet riding a motorcycle is to have responsible riding habits, professional training, and the required protective gear

111—ADRENAL INSUFFICIENCY: ACUTE AND FULMINANT

The adrenal glands are located close to the upper pole of both kidneys and produce hormones that are essential for survival. Each gland has two portions: the central one is called medullary, and the outer section is called cortical. The former produces cathecolamines, epinephrine (adrenalin), and norepinephrine. The latter manufactures steroids. Insufficient levels of adrenal hormones in the circulating blood results from "adrenal insufficiency."

TYPES OF ADRENAL INSUFFICIENCY

There are three types:

- *Primary adrenal insufficiency.* This is caused by anatomic destruction of the adrenal glands. Decades ago, tuberculosis was the most frequent cause. Currently, in the United States, an immune reaction is responsible for the majority of cases. It is called Addison's disease
- *Secondary adrenal insufficiency.* The pituitary gland is diseased and does not produce enough ACTH, a hormone that stimulates steroids production by the adrenal gland, or it may also be caused by the use of steroids for chronic diseases. When for some reason the patient stops taking them, the adrenal gland is too lazy to manufacture the hormone and that may lead to an adrenal crisis
- *Acute adrenal insufficiency.* This is an exacerbation of chronic adrenal insufficiency, usually provoked by surgery, anesthesia, dehydration, trauma, asthma, stress, hypothermia, alcohol, myocardial infarction, fever, sepsis, pain, hypoglycemia, psychosis or depression, exogenous steroid withdrawal

A crisis of acute adrenal insufficiency can be fatal.

SYMPTOMS OF ADRENAL INSUFFICIENCY

These are nonspecific: weakness, skin pigmentation, and weight loss are the most frequent. Other symptoms are abdominal pain, salt craving, diarrhea, constipation, fainting.

TREATMENT OF AN ADRENAL INSUFFICIENCY CRISIS

- Immediate hospitalization in the intensive care unit
- Maintenance of the circulation, breathing, and airway
- Correction of hypoglycemia, low serum sodium, high levels of calcium and potassium
- Administration of hydrocortisone and fludrocortisone
- Treatment of the underlying problem that precipitated the crisis
- Consultation with endocrinologist

PRESIDENT JOHN F. KENNEDY AND HIS ADDISON'S DISEASE

He suffered from the disease but kept it secret. According to medical records released in 2000, John F. Kennedy was diagnosed Addison's disease in 1947. He was a sick man for the rest of his life. By the time he was president, he was on ten to twelve different medications, antispasmodics and paregoric for his bowels, muscular relaxants, phenobarbital, Librium, meprobamate, codeine, Demerol, methadone, oral cortisone, injectable cortisone, testosterone, and Nembutal. As if all of that wasn't enough, he had a disabling low back pain, several unsuccessful surgeries for this condition, and there were times when the White House physician had to inject novocaine in his lower spine area six times a day. He also had compression fractures of the spine and osteoporosis. At times he was on crutches.

112—ADVANCED AGE

Timely diagnosis and treatment can make you younger.

THE SEARCH FOR ABNORMALITIES

It doesn't take more than a few minutes to examine a patient at the office and detect life-threatening cardiovascular abnormalities.

Elderly patients are prone to develop cardiovascular disorders. This happens because the heart and arteries suffer a natural deterioration and also because the person's body was mistreated with many years of smoking, booze, junk food, neglected hypertension and cholesterol levels, scant physical activity, chronic stress due to financial hardships, loneliness, or a marriage that lives in a war zone, a costly divorce, or problems with the children who are no longer children. You name it. People have it!

So it is not surprising to see elderly patients having not only heart disease but involvement of other vascular territories. Sometimes, individuals who are happy also develop cardiovascular disorders, their bodies are plagued by disease, and they never had a single major complaint.

I recently saw a seventy-year-old man referred to us for a "routine" examination. He felt "excellent" and was playing golf three times a week. He thought that there was nothing wrong with him. In that examination I discovered he had severe blockages of his coronary arteries, critical carotid artery disease, and a large abdominal aortic aneurysm. He said, "Doc, are you kidding me? I really feel great!" That evening he was admitted to the hospital. He had quadruple coronary bypass and carotid endarterectomy (surgery to relieve the carotid obstruction) the same day. A few days later, he had a successful resection of his abdominal aortic aneurysm.

CARDIOVASCULAR EXAMINATION THAT MAY DISCLOSE THE NEED FOR QUICK INTERVENTION

Neck

The **carotid arteries** run at both sides of the neck. These display a pulsation felt by the examiner's finger. A weak pulsation suggests that the carotid artery might be narrower than normal due to an atherosclerotic plaque. An obese neck may yield a poor pulsation because of the fatty tissue interposed between the artery and the examining thumb. Total absence of the carotid pulsation invites the exclusion of a complete blockage.

The stethoscope applied in the neck searches for a bruit. A bruit is a "blowing" sound caused by the turbulence of the blood that gets across a partially blocked artery. An ultrasound of the carotids will detect obstructive lesions. If more details are required, a MRA (magnetic resonance angiogram) is obtained.

Severe carotid stenosis (stenosis means blockage) may require stent treatment or surgery. These modalities of treatment may prevent a catastrophic stroke.

Heart

Coronary Arteries

Are these blocked by atherosclerotic plaques, and if so, how much? The symptoms you describe are extremely important: chest pain or tightness, shortness of breath, and others. Some people have severe coronary artery disease and never had any cardiac symptoms, and if they did, they thought these were not due to heart disease. Occasionally, an electrocardiogram shows previous myocardial infarctions, and the patient is totally surprised about this finding. Acute myocardial infarctions then can be silent or unrecognized: "I have occasional indigestion," which at times is truly an expression of coronary artery disease.

A myocardial infarction may also occur during the sleep. The patient wakes up in the morning, has her/his usual breakfast, and goes to work. A year later, she or he is told that her routine electrocardiogram showed an unequivocal evidence of a previous myocardial infarction.

Treatment approach varies a great deal: when the coronary blockages are not severe, the patient is treated with medications and lifestyle changes. If the arterial obstructions are severe, they are relieved by balloon angioplasty, usually followed by stent placement. When the arterial obstructions cannot be negotiated, bypass surgery may be required.

Heart Valves

The most characteristic valve abnormality that can cause sudden death is **aortic stenosis.** The aortic valve accumulates calcium over the years, and at one point, the valve opening is so small that the blood ejected by the left ventricle can barely get through it.

The diagnosis of severe aortic stenosis is suspected by listening to the chest with a stethoscope, and this shows a typical murmur. The diagnosis is corroborated by an echocardiogram. Replacement of the aortic valve is generally carried out. A cardiac catheterization is done preoperatively to see if, in addition to valve replacement, coronary bypass is also needed.

Aortic valvular insufficiency. The valve is unable to close normally, and that results in regurgitation of blood from the aorta back into the left ventricle. When it is severe, valve replacement becomes a serious consideration. *Acute mitral insufficiency* can also be life-threatening by causing acute pulmonary edema.

The Myocardium

A weak heart muscle may be the result of many different causes, viral infections, coronary artery disease, alcohol, hypertension, valvular heart disease, and many others.

The usual measure of the left ventricular pumping function, namely, its capacity to eject blood every time it contracts is called the ejection fraction. This is the percentage of blood thrown into the arterial system with each heartbeat. Normally it is 50% to 75%. **A severe reduction of the EF to 35% or less predisposes to sudden death.** In addition to medications for heart failure, an automatic defibrillator is often implanted.

The heart's electrical system. The heart has an electrical system that generates its own current and transmits it through the so-called conducting system. This consists of a series of bundles widespread in the cardiac muscle. The electrical current stimulates the heart muscle, and this results in its contraction.

This electrical circuit may suffer from blockages, interruptions, short circuits, battery failure, and other disturbances that lead to abnormalities of the cardiac rhythm (arrhythmias).

There are different types of arrhythmias. Some are benign. Others are malignant and may lead to a cardiac arrest.

A cardiac arrest may result from very slow or very fast heart rates.

Treatment is provided with drugs, pacemakers, ablation, or intracardiac defibrillators. Some cardiologists subspecialize in electrophysiology, and their expertise is at times required to provide optimal antiarrhythmic therapy.

ABDOMINAL AORTIC ANEURYSM (AAA)

Please see section 1.

RISK OF FALLING

Millions of seniors fall, at times, with dreadful consequences. As many as 40% of adults over age 65 fall each year in the United States, and in people over age 75, falls cause 70% of all accidental deaths.

Clinical observation indicates that many older patients do not have adequate protection to prevent disabling or fatal falls.

Advancing age, housebound status, and living alone are common risk factors that lead to falls. Other factors contributing to falls are dizzy spells, medical conditions that affect gait and balance, a long list of medications that slow down the heart rate or the blood pressure to levels that are not well tolerated. Bending over or standing up may produce blood pressure fluctuations resulting in severe dizziness.

Cerebrovascular insufficiency and inner ear dysfunction may produce vertigo. Those who have experienced vertigo know how disabling and scary it can be. Everything spins and if the patient is standing he or she will land on the ground fast. Even while lying down vertigo is a frightening experience. Poor vision doesn't help either.

Severe arthritis of lumbar spine, hips, and knees; calluses; prominent bunions; and ulcers impair the patient's gait, and falls are common. Diffused muscular atrophy due to advanced age and no regular exercise weakens the muscles of the lower extremities, and some falls are almost inevitable.

Alcohol consumption in the elderly is often underestimated or forgotten.

Recommended routine tests in individuals at risk for falling include complete blood count; serum sodium, magnesium, and potassium levels; blood urea nitrogen, creatinine, glucose, vitamin B12, and thyroid function tests. In cases of head injury, a CT or a MRI of the brain may be necessary.

113—AIDS

Acquired immunodeficiency syndrome (AIDS) usually has prolonged, nonspecific symptoms such as fever, night sweats, weight loss, and easy fatigability. Occasionally, it runs a brutally aggressive course, and in hours or a few days the patient is gone. Those who suffer from this disorder may have a cardiac arrest that results from AIDS cardiomyopathy or develop an accelerated course of severe respiratory failure due to fulminant pneumonia, typically produced by the *Pneumocystis carinii*.

A forty-five-year-old patient requested an urgent office appointment because she had cough and fever. She was a medical doctor who had originally been a man, but years prior she had undergone extensive surgery to become a woman. That is defined as a transsexual person. Her husband of about the same age accompanied her. The vagina had been surgically created with a segment of bowel that did not allow for penile penetration. The couple regularly practiced anal sex. She appeared acutely ill, had severe shortness of breath and was immediately hospitalized. She had AIDS, extensive Pneumocystis carinii *pneumonia, and died in forty-eight hours. Her husband died of AIDS complications too six months later.*

**

Another case: Charlie, a thirty-year-old homosexual male nurse developed fever, cough, quick prostration, and respiratory embarrassment. He realized he was going to die fast. He had extensive Pneumocystis carinii *pneumonia and refractory respiratory failure. He was fully alert. One day before he died, he instructed his sister on the suit, shirt, tie, and shoes he wanted to be dressed at his funeral.*

Who can forget cases like these?

114—AIR BAG FATALITIES

The National Highway Traffic Safety Administration reported that from 1990 to the year 2000, 6,377 lives were saved and numerous injuries prevented due to the protection offered by air bags. Occasionally, something goes wrong with air bags, and fatalities have occurred from their deployment: in the lapse of 10 years, 176 fatalities occurred—104 were children and 71 adults.

CHILDREN

Infants placed in the front seat of a car in a rear-facing child seat have accounted for 19 deaths. This way of placing a child in a car carries significant risks because of the proximity of the child's head to the compartment where the air bag is housed. When an air bag deploys, it does it at a speed of 200 miles per hour. The child's head may undergo serious injury. Other children are placed in the front seat but looking forward. If the child is not restrained, trouble is expected. Children who died were not restrained or improperly restrained. The best way to restrain children under 40 lbs is a booster seat in the back seat.

ADULTS

Most of air bag fatalities in adults are due to failure to use a safety belt. Those who were properly restrained and died were small-sized females who were positioned too close to the steering wheel.

Adult and children safety belt laws and their enforcement will lead to increased safety.

My wife Cristina was driving her car and crossing an intersection. A man driving without a license dismissed a stop sign and hit her vehicle badly. Her air bag functioned immediately, but it caught fire. She was trapped by a safety belt that she couldn't release. The man responsible for the accident helped her to come out of the car. She had some injuries but recovered.

As you can appreciate, air bags may fail to protect you because of (a) failure to deploy or (b) defective deployment.

For more information, contact the following:

Air Bag & Seat Belt Safety Campaign, National Safety Council, 1025 Conn. Ave., NW, Suite 1200, Washington DC 20036, 202-625-2570

National Safety Council, 1121 Spring Lake Drive, Itasca, IL, 60143-3201, voice: 630-285-1121

115—ANABOLIC STEROIDS

Illicit use of androgens has been a recognized problem among competitive athletes and body builders. It's been estimated that over 1 million persons had previous use of steroids. Anabolic steroids such as testosterone, stanozolol, and nandrolone are frequently used in combination at high doses for periods of weeks to months. **These high doses commonly exceed 100 times the doses used to treat medical conditions.**

There are reports in the medical literature of young men age less than thirty-five who developed severe coronary atherosclerosis, myocardial infarctions, and strokes attributed to the excessive use of anabolic steroids.

116—ANAPHYLAXIS—ACUTE ALLERGIC REACTION

Anaphylaxis is a serious and rapid allergic reaction that involves several parts of the body. **An anaphylactic crisis demands immediate recognition since death may occur minutes to hours after the first symptoms.**

This reaction appears seconds to minutes after administration of a specific offender, called antigen, that enters the body, generally by injection, and less commonly, by ingestion. The body manufactures the wrong kind of antibody, called immunoglobulin E (IgE). The IgE sticks to cells in our bodies (mast cells, basophils), which release substances that cause the bronchial tubes to constrict and the arterial system to dilate. Histamine is one of these substances.

Anaphylaxis usually presents with severe respiratory distress followed by vascular collapse. The former occurs because acute swelling of the tongue blocks the airway, laryngeal edema (swelling of the larynx is described as a lump in the throat), or wheezing due to bronchial spasm or constriction, associated with a feeling of tightness in the chest, or a combination of all of the above. Vascular collapse is due to vasodilatation of the body vessels, which causes a drastic blood pressure drop.

SOME SUBSTANCES THAT ARE CAPABLE OF PRODUCING AN ANAPHYLACTIC REACTION

Food. Eggs, seafood, nuts, grains, beans, chocolate, bananas, avocados, kiwi fruit, figs, and other fruits and vegetables, including potatoes and tomatoes

Occupational products (occupational proteins). Mainly in rubber latex gloves, catheters, other medical products. All these are mainly used by health care workers (nurses)

Insects. Wasp, bees, ants

Pollen extracts. ragweed, grass, trees

Proteins in the form of hormones. Example: insulin

Drugs. Most commonly **antibiotics,** such as penicillin, cephalosporins, amphotericin B, nitrofurantoin, local anesthetics (procaine, lidocaine), vitamins (thiamine, folic acid), diagnostic agents, occupational chemicals (ethylene oxide), aspirin and other pain killers (called NSAIDs)

Careful with beta-blockers. These medications are used for heart disease (coronary heart disease, heart failure, arrhythmias), hypertension, familial tremor, migraine headaches, and glaucoma. Mild allergic reactions may become severe in people taking these medications.

Exercise. It may precipitate an anaphylactic reaction and so may exercise after eating food. This is called **exercise-induced food-dependent anaphylaxis.**

Unknown. When the cause of the anaphylactic reaction is unknown, it is called **idiopathic.** This has been thought to be due to a disturbance of certain body cells called "mast cells" that cause them to release histamine and other chemicals with a similar action.

CLINICAL MANIFESTATIONS OF ANAPHYLAXIS

Anaphylaxis can cause the following:

- An itchy rash (hives or urticaria)
- Swelling or angioedema (sometimes it affects the eyelids and the tissues around the eyes are markedly swollen)
- Swelling of the tongue and throat causing difficulty in swallowing or breathing
- Wheezing with asthmatic attack
- Vomiting
- Abdominal cramps
- Death that results from obstruction to breathing or very severe low blood pressure (anaphylactic shock)

THE BEST TREATMENT FOR ANAPHYLAXIS

Adrenaline (epinephrine) is the standard treatment for life-threatening anaphylactic reactions. It is given by injection, intravenously, intramuscularly, or subcutaneously.

For adult, 0.3 mg and for child, 0.15 mg. There are special adrenalin kits.

If you are a candidate for anaphylactic reactions, **take the adrenalin kit with you at all times and wherever you go.**

Make sure you check the expiration date on the syringe and replace it on time. It can lose effectiveness if you let it go out of date. Some manufacturers will let you know when the time comes to replace the kit.

Follow storage instructions and never place an adrenaline syringe in the freezer. When the adrenaline solution is becoming useless, it may change its color to yellow or brown, but don't count on it. Weaker adrenaline may maintain the same color.

The administration of adrenaline carries its own risk. It may cause serious cardiac arrhythmias, and in cardiac or sensitive patients, it may even lead to a cardiac arrest. Adrenaline is a wonderful lifesaving drug, and you'll be able to appreciate that by reading some of my patients' experiences with this drug a few lines below. However, **you need specific instructions by your doctor about the right dose to use in case of an emergency, on when, how, and where to inject it** (muscle, body fat under the skin, intravenously in special cases), whether or not the injection could be repeated in 20 minutes, and for how long you should be under careful medical observation after the initial attack has receded.

In some cases there's a second allergic reaction that takes place hours after the first one. At least 6 hours of medical observation is necessary.

The following stories belong to three patients of mine who developed acute anaphylactic reactions and survived. One of them occurred unexpectedly in the intensive care unit. The other two happened outside the hospital.

When I was a teenager, I read the famous Scottish writer Stevenson's novella about the strange case of Dr. Jekyll and Mr. Hyde and also saw a movie about that story where the former drinks a liquid mixture he had created and suffers impressive physical changes in his face—and soul—in a few seconds. That was the case of the man and the beast as the author had described.

This story made an impact on me and never forgot it. Many years later, as a practicing cardiologist, while making my rounds in the ICU of St. Francis Hospital, Miami Beach, I saw one of my elderly patients, Harry, returning to the ICU in a stretcher after having an intravenous iodine injection in the radiology department for a kidney test.

He looked fine. He was a happy man. Always showing a smile so big that extended from one earlobe to the other.

We saw each other, and he raised his hand to say hello to me. I did the same. All of a sudden his face began to experience the most rapid and impressive changes. His eyelids, forehead, and his lips got swollen. I saw his tongue getting bigger in seconds. So big that his tongue blocked his mouth entirely. His face turned blue, his eyes bulged in despair. He couldn't catch his breath.

Luckily, I was there to assist him right away and so was an anesthesiologist. He was intubated (a tube was placed into his trachea) and responded to an injection of adrenaline.

He was saved because he had immediate medical attention. If his reaction had occurred in the elevator or the hospital corridors while being transported back to the ICU from the radiology department, most likely he would have died.

**

A urologist and his wife went to Paris for a "second honeymoon." The first night in the hotel was supposed to be all-romance-and-champagne celebration. While in the hotel room, he suddenly had a choking sensation and was unable to breathe. Since he had a history of severe allergic reactions, he and his wife had been instructed to inject him adrenaline, in case of emergency.

Well, now they had the emergency. She gave it to him immediately in the arm and in a few minutes resolved the crisis. He told me: "Ed, if I had not had my adrenaline syringe with me at the time, I would have died. It was terrible. I just couldn't breathe!"

**

Years ago, I examined a Vietnam veteran in a VA outpatient facility for a routine examination. He was fifty-five and in general good health although twenty years prior he had had a foot infection treated with an antibiotic and had an acute anaphylactic reaction that was controlled by an adrenalin injection.

*Although he had never had another allergic reaction in two decades, I urged him not to leave the clinic without an adrenalin kit. He didn't want to bother with it. I insisted and got the kit for him that day and strongly recommended him to carry it on **permanent basis.***

*A month later he came to the office just to say hello and give me his "thanks." I asked him: "Thanks for what?" This was the reason: The day he had his physical examination with me, one month prior, he had gotten the adrenalin syringe that he didn't want to bother with, and **that evening** he had a severe acute allergic reaction, and the adrenaline shot saved him.*

117—ANESTHESIA

General anesthesia if often accompanied by high blood pressure and a rapid pulse (tachycardia). Although this may be due to an incomplete anesthesia, more commonly these abnormalities are related to withdrawal from antihypertensive medications, low oxygen concentration in the blood (hypoxemia), delirium, or bladder distension. These changes require specific treatment to avoid additional complications.

General anesthesia is generally safe but not always safe. There are medical conditions that may predispose to life-threatening arrhythmias. There are medications provided during anesthesia that may protect the patient from having serious rhythm problems or predispose him/her to them. The anesthesiologist must be pharmacologically sophisticated to deal with this delicate situation. A consultation with a cardiologist and the availability of this specialist during anesthesia is highly recommended.

The conditions that require special attention are the following:

* Congenital QT interval (see section106)
* Brugada syndrome (see section 101)
* Wolf-Parkinson-White (WPW) syndrome (see section 109)
* Arrhythmogenic right ventricular dysplasia (ARVD) (see section 100)
* Coronary artery disease (see section 87)
* Cardiomyopathy (see section 70-92)
* Myocarditis (see section 120)
* Patients known to have intermittent life-threatening arrhythmias

Shivering is a phenomenon that may occur as a result of hypothermia or the action of a volatile anesthetic. The trouble with shivering is that it increases oxygen consumption. Patients with cardiovascular disease do not tolerate the consequences of shivering well. The drug meperidine (Demerol) in low dose controls the shivering pretty well although it isn't known how it does it.

Post-operative complications seen after general anesthesia are frequent in patients with risk factors. Some of them are the following:

• Myocardial infarction
• Heart failure
• Malignant arrhythmias

- High catecholamine levels
- Drug effects
- Anemia
- Low blood volume
- Increased coagulability of the blood
- Cardiac death

All general anesthetic and the techniques used to apply them are potentially capable of producing serious complications. This is particularly true for cardiovascular patients.

It is essential to proceed with a good preoperative evaluation, monitor the patient thoroughly during and following anesthesia, and select the anesthetic appropriate for the planned surgical procedure.

Recently, Michael Jackson died from a combination of the general anesthetic propofol and the anti-anxiety drug lorazepam. His personal physician administered 25 milligrams of propofol diluted with lidocaine shortly before Jackson's death.

There are reports of self-administration of propofol for recreational purposes. Short-term effects include euphoria, hallucinations, and disinhibition. Propofol is particularly dangerous without proper medical monitoring and at least three deaths from self-administration have been recorded.

118—ANOREXIA NERVOSA

This is a psychiatric disorder that most commonly occurs in women younger than twenty-five years of age.

Normal people get pleasure from eating. Patients suffering from anorexia derive pleasure from not eating. Sometimes, they throw food out instead of eating it. They have a distorted body image, and when they have lost lots of weight and are only left with skin and bones, they still feel they are too fat. They usually (and secretly) take laxatives, diuretics, amphetamines, or induce vomiting.

The cause of the disease is unknown. These patients are active, alert, and may be exercise fanatics. They also tend to deny they are ill.

Sometimes hospitalization is necessary to provide hyperalimentation with intravenous solutions and psychiatric treatment.

Many of these people recover with appropriate management, but the condition must be followed closely. One out of 20 patients die from it.

119—APPENDICITIS

The appendix is a little pouch that projects out from the colon on the lower right side of the abdomen. Nobody ever discovered what is the reason for its existence. But this much is certain: when food waste or a piece of stool becomes trapped in this tiny organ, it becomes infected and causes acute appendicitis. When the appendix perforates, its contents, full of germs are drained into the peritoneal cavity. That means acute peritonitis, and very serious trouble.

Appendicitis most often affects persons between the ages of ten and thirty, but younger and older people may suffer from acute appendicitis. This disease is one of the most frequent emergencies requiring surgical treatment in children. Advanced age is not immune to it. I once had a patient aged eighty with this condition.

Children are more likely to have a ruptured appendix than adults are. The main symptom is abdominal pain around the navel first, but later on, it moves to the belly's lower right quadrant and settles there. In 6-12 hours the pain increases in severity. Since the appendix's anatomical position varies from patient to patient, sometimes, the location of the pain is not as typical as described.

When the doctor examines the abdomen and presses his/her hand over the lower right quadrant, pain increases but more so when the hand is released. This is because there is a little rebound of the peritoneal membrane touching the appendix.

Acute appendicitis may mimic other conditions such as ectopic pregnancy, ovarian cyst, kidney stone, and inflammatory disease of the bowel.

Clinical experience by the health care practitioner is important to diagnose appendicitis. An abdominal x-ray or ultrasound may be recommended by your doctor but more commonly a computerized tomography (CT) scan is used to confirm the diagnosis. Once acute appendicitis is diagnosed, surgery must be performed quickly. The surgeon may choose laparoscopic approach, which requires a small abdominal incision. A little pencil-like tube is inserted through the abdomen. It has its own light and video camera with a system that magnifies the size of intra-abdominal anatomy, and tiny instruments are used to remove the appendix.

If the appendix ruptures the condition becomes more serious. There's peritonitis, and a laparoscopic technique is no longer applicable. A larger and open abdominal incision is required so the surgeon can clean the abdominal cavity from the abundance of germs it contains.

The famous magician Harry Houdini, who also was a brilliant stunt performer and escapologist, couldn't escape from a perforated appendix and the resulting peritonitis. He died on October 26, 1926. He thought his abdominal pains had resulted from the fist blows that someone had delivered to his abdomen as part of a show a few days prior. By the time the diagnosis of peritonitis was made, it was too late to save his life.

Peritonitis without surgical treatment is generally fatal.

120—ASTHMA

The wheezing alarm goes off.

Asthma is predominantly an outpatient condition and affects about 2.5% of the population. Many people suffer from mild to moderate asthma and are able to control the disease. At times, asthma shows an ugly face, and can be lethal.

How often asthma is fatal is uncertain since an unknown number of patients succumb before reaching the hospital.

The disease is characterized by bronchial constriction (also called bronchospasm). The bronchial tubes become obstructed, and the air passage is severely affected.

WHAT MAKES AN ASTHMA ATTACK FATAL?

An acute asthma attack is a particularly serious event when it is associated with altered state of consciousness or respiratory arrest. This is more so when the patient has been receiving adequate therapy and develops a very severe sudden asthmatic attack.

Asthma sudden death may occur through two mechanisms: (1) ventilatory failure and respiratory arrest, and (2) cardiac arrest (it results from ventilatory failure).

Ventilatory failure is the result of progressive increase in airway resistance and resistance to conventional asthmatic therapy. Cardiac arrest may occur during severe asthma in association with severe respiratory failure. Some sudden deaths were reported in association with the administration of excessive use of pressurized aerosols or myocardial ischemia (deficient heart muscle blood supply) due to an excessive doses of isoproterenol or other beta-adrenergic medications employed to relieve bronchospasm.

Respiratory acidosis or significant accumulation of carbon dioxide due to respiratory failure is an indicator of potentially life-threatening arrhythmias. This condition is diagnosed by the routine analysis of arterial blood gases.

The acute mental and physical stress of a very severe asthmatic attack is capable of inducing lethal cardiac arrhythmias too.

WHAT CAUSES ACUTE ASTHMATIC DECOMPENSATION?

Bronchial constriction is at the crux of the problem in asthma. Some patients do not have mucous plugging or mucosa edema of the airways, whereas others fill their airways with mucous and have extensive inflammation.

SOME CHARACTERISTIC FEATURES THAT INDICATE ASTHMA MAY BE LIFE-THREATENING

- Increasing wheeze and breathlessness. Patient unable to complete sentences in one breath or unable to get up from a chair or bed
- Respiratory rate of 25 breaths/minute and persistent tachycardia (heart rate acceleration)
- Abnormal peak expiratory flow

IMMINENT LIFE-THREATENING SIGNS

Any of the following indicates a very severe asthma crisis

- Cyanosis (blue face, lips, and hands)

- Bradycardia (slow pulse)
- Exhaustion
- Confusion
- Unconsciousness
- Silent chest on auscultation (replaced previous wheezing)
- Sometimes patients who do not have these dangerous warning features also may develop critical asthma and present with an attack that appears to be mild

IMPORTANT FEATURES THAT SIGNAL A GREATER LIKELIHOOD OF FATAL ASTHMA

- Age—younger people are more prone to life-threatening events
- Previous life-threatening exacerbations, hospital admission within the past year
- Inadequate management
- Lack of access to a medical facility

PRECIPITATING FACTORS

- Air pollution
- Allergens (substances capable of producing allergic reactions)
- Respiratory infections
- Air pollution
- Weather changes
- Medications (aspirin, beta-blockers, nonsteroidal anti-inflammatory drugs) have been shown to precipitate near fatal or fatal asthmatic attack
- Severe stress and emotional upsets have led to acute asphyxia

TREATMENT AND PREVENTION

Initial treatment of the asthmatic attack varies from country to country although there is agreement on this: mechanical ventilation with the introduction of a tube in the trachea (endotracheal intubation) should be avoided if possible.

Large doses of b2-agonists (medications that produce bronchial expansion) and intravenous steroids (these reduce bronchial mucosa inflammation) must be used. The respiratory function needs to be monitored by an expert.

After discharge from the hospital, the patient must be monitored closely. If a recurrence occurs, he or she should have a rapid admission to a specialized care unit. Action plans need to be carefully structured.

A major cause of near fatal or fatal asthmatic attacks is the patient's and/or the physician's failure to recognize or underestimate the severity of an asthma attack.

High-risk patients need to be timely identified, and treatment should be provided by a very knowledgeable health care practitioner.

121—BEE AND WASP STING

Those who are particularly sensitive to stinging insect venom may have a very serious reaction, which at times is fatal. This applies to bees, wasps, hornets, bumblebees, and ants.

In the United States, approximately 100 people die each year from sting reactions. These insects cause more deaths than from spiders or snakes bites. From 100 persons who get stung by insects, one doesn't survive.

The initial reaction is "local," and the skin show redness, pain and swelling, and at times, itching. It lasts for a few hours, and when it disappears is good news. Sometimes, the local reaction is more severe and lasts several days. That is not a major problem either. The trouble—and sometimes, the drama unfolds if there's a generalized allergic reaction: the blood pressure drops, and the bronchial tubes constrict. Please, see section 116. The patient experiences stomach cramps and diarrhea, itching around the eyes, shortness of breath, wheezing, loss of consciousness, drastic fall in the blood pressure, and collapse. These reactions occur in 5-30 minutes.

THE SENSITIVITY ISSUE

The more quickly the reaction develops, the more serious the consequences. Sometimes, the first time a person is stung does not have a reaction, but antibodies are produced and if another sting occurs in the future, the insect venom combines with the antibody and causes a mess of unprecedented proportions, such as the symptoms and events I described in the preceding paragraph.

STINGS

When the insect stings, it takes 2-3 minutes for the venom sac to inject all of it. So if the stinger is removed right away, the reaction will be less severe. Honeybees have a barbed stinger. Only this insect leaves the stinger with its venom sac attached in the skin of its victim. **Never use the thumb and forefinger or tweezers to remove the stinger. This maneuver forces more venom from the sac into the wound.**

PREVENTION

- Call a pest control operator to spray the patio, picnic, garbage areas, and nests. You could use yourself commercially available stinging insect control aerosols, but you'll be safer with a professional exterminator
- If you are outdoors, keep food covered until eaten, especially soft drinks and ripe fruit. Bees and wasps like the smell of BBQ as much as you do. They are very attracted to it
- If a bee or a wasp gets into a moving car, don't show any signs of distress. The insect badly wants to get out of the vehicle. Don't try to hit it. Just open the window and allow the insect to escape
- Perfume, hair spray, suntan lotion, aftershave lotion, soaps, shampoos should be avoided. Wear a hat and closed shoes. Avoid bright clothes: they attract insects
- Additional precautions: wear a head veil, long sleeves, pant legs tucked into boots
- Hypersensitive persons should never be alone when hiking, swimming, boating, golfing, fishing, or during other outdoors activities. It is advisable for them to use a Medic Alert tag that can be purchased at the Medic Alert Foundation, 2323 Colorado Avenue, Turlock, California 95380 at telephone number 1-800-922-3320
- Highly sensitive persons should have two emergency kits prescribed for them by their physician and have easy access to them at all times. One should be carried at all times, and the other should be kept in the family car. The kit should contain one sterile syringe of epinephrine (adrenalin), an antihistamine, one tourniquet, and alcohol sponges. Insect sting kits are sold in pharmacies by prescription
- Those who have experienced a reaction to insect stings are recommended to consult an allergist. They undergo skin testing and are desensitized with a series of appropriate venous injections

122—BLUNT CHEST TRAUMA

Chest trauma is a significant cause of mortality in the United States. Blunt injury to the thorax affects any one or all components of the chest wall or bony skeleton (ribs, clavicles, scapulae, sternum) or organs located inside the thoracic cavity (lungs, pleurae, trachea, bronchial tubes, esophagus, heart, aorta, pericardium and pulmonary vessels, and the diaphragm, the muscle that separates the chest cavity from the abdominal cavity).

Trauma is the leading cause of death, hospitalization, and disability in Americans aged 1-55 years. It kills 100,000 people annually in the United States. Blunt thoracic injuries are directly responsible for 20-25% of all trauma deaths.

By far, the most important cause of serious blunt chest trauma is motor vehicle accidents (MVAs), which account for 70-80% of this kind of injury. Pedestrians struck by vehicles, violent acts, and falls are additional causes.

INJURIES THAT RESULT FROM BLUNT THORACIC TRAUMA

The pain associated with rib fractures makes breathing difficult. Lung perforation with pneumothorax (collapse of the lung due to the entrance of air in the pleural space) and blood in the pleural space (hemothorax) may also impair oxygenation.

Cardiac chamber rupture or severe injuries to the aorta or pulmonary artery usually result in death before treatment can be provided. This happens because of rapid exsanguination that causes irreversible shock.

123—BOTULISM

This is a life-threatening disease caused by toxins produced by a germ called *Clostridium botulinum*. This word has its roots in the Latin word *botulus* that means sausage. In the nineteenth century, eating sausage was a lethal sport. A sausage is something that raises fear and suspicion under normal circumstances. Now, imagine how dangerous it was over a century ago, when sausage meat was rotten due to poor hygiene conditions and no refrigeration.

Botulism is one of the most powerful known poisons, and it is absorbed in the stomach and the colon. Although home-canned foods with putrid odor are the most frequently implicated vehicle, **foods that contain these germs may look and taste normal.** You may be wondering how it is possible that foul-smelling food is consumed by some people.

Contamination is also helped by insufficiently heated food because the toxin is not destroyed. Heat does it. The foods most frequently affected are fish and fish products, relish, and chili peppers.

The incubation period of this disease, namely, the time that goes from the food consumption and the first clinical manifestations of the disease is 18-36 hours. Then, trouble starts: one eyelid drops (ptosis), and vision becomes blurred. This is followed by paralysis of facial muscles, tongue, palate, larynx, diaphragm, and intercostal muscles (muscles located in between ribs).

HOW IS THE DIAGNOSIS OF BOTULISM MADE?

Usual laboratory tests are useless. The most sensitive diagnostic test remains the injection of the patient's serum intraperitoneally to mice. If the patient has botulism, the animals will die in 24-48 hours. This is carried out in health departments of CDC in Atlanta, Georgia.

TREATMENT

- Respiratory failure quickly appears and may require endotracheal intubation (a tube inserted in the trachea through the nose or the mouth) and respiratory support by a respirator for days to months. A tracheostomy (a hole done in anterior neck to create a tracheal opening) may be required
- The disease must be reported to the authorities
- Trivalent botulism antitoxin type ABE must be injected (Connaught Laboratories, Swiftwater, Pennsylvania)

PREVENTION

- Boiling food destroys the toxin
- For those who work in laboratories with botulism toxins, there's a vaccine called pentavalent botulism vaccine

BOTULISM IN CHILDREN

This disease was not recognized up until 1976. There are 30-80 cases in the United States annually. Ninety percent of these cases occur in children less than 6 months of age. Honey may be contaminated, and this is found in 10% of honey samples.

It is recommended that children less than 12 months old not ingest honey.

When botulism attacks a child, an eyelid may drop, he/she becomes floppy and lethargic. Other symptoms vary from constipation to sudden death.

124—CARDIOVASCULAR RISK FACTORS NEGLECT AND/OR IGNORANCE

Cardiovascular disease (CVD) is a major cause of suffering, disability, and death.

Sudden cardiac death (SCD) occurs in individuals who suffer from various forms of heart disease, involving the coronary arteries, the heart muscle, cardiac valves, congenital heart disease, arrhythmias, or pericardial tamponade. Infrequently, but particularly shocking, is the SCD that occurs when there's no recognizable evidence of heart disease. Another ugly surprise occurs when a relatively minor contusion of the chest hits the thorax during a highly vulnerable period of the cardiac cycle and causes a deadly ventricular fibrillation (commotion cordis).

So as you can see, life can be tricky and unfair, and lives can certainly be lost because of situations that are beyond our control. Having said that, I have no hesitation to tell you that many individuals cut their lives short because of ignorance and neglect.

400,000 people die annually in the United States because of smoking. These demises are totally preventable. The use and abuse of unhealthy foods that children and adults consume with such a pleasure constantly create pipelines that end in intensive care units or funeral homes.

In my daily practice, I see patients who have mercilessly damaged their cardiovascular system during decades of poor eating habits, lack of physical activity, uncontrolled hypertension, serum lipids abnormalities and diabetes, smoking, stress, chronic depression and unhappiness, obesity, and other CVRF.

It's been estimated that in 2007 there were approximately 79 million Americans (one out of 4 persons) who had some form of cardiovascular disease. Recent statistics show that 38.5% of deaths in the United States is attributable to CVD.

CVD is responsible for more U.S. deaths than the next five leading causes of death combined. CVD remains the number one killer of both men and women in the United States and other Western countries. In China and other Asian countries, CV mortality is two—to fivefold higher than infectious disease mortality.

SOME CARDIOVASCULAR RISK FACTORS

* Poor information on health issues
* Neglect of learned health issues
* Cigarette smoking
* Hypertension or elevated blood pressure
* Elevated serum total cholesterol levels
* Low serum high-density lipoprotein (HDL)
* High levels of homocysteine
* Diabetes
* Advanced age
* Obesity
* Abdominal obesity
* Morbid obesity
* Chronic infections such as periodontitis (gum infection)
* Chronic inflammatory illnesses
* Severe depression
* Psychiatric illness
* Personality disorders
* Severe stress
* Prolonged physical inactivity or sedentary lifestyle
* Excessive alcohol consumption
* Gestational diabetes
* Family history of heart disease, hypertension, diabetes, or high lipids levels
* C-reactive protein elevated blood levels

In order to grasp the immensity of the CVD problem and what this entitles, please review in contents part 1 and part 4, and you'll see a profuse number of cardiovascular conditions. Here, we'll place emphasis on the illnesses that result from atherosclerosis and hypertension since they are more prevalent in our society.

1—Myocardial infarction
    Angina pectoris
    Heart failure
    Hypertension
    Coronary death

2—Cerebrovascular disease (CVD) and carotid artery disease (CAD)
    Stroke and TIA (transient ischemic attacks)

3—Peripheral vascular disease (PVD)
    Blockages of arteries of lower extremities (intermittent claudication: this means pain in calves, thighs, or buttocks during walking due to deficient blood supply to the muscles of these areas
    Aortic aneurysm (thoracic or abdominal)

UNAVOIDABLE CVRF

Certain factors you cannot avoid no matter what you do: race (Afro Americans have higher incidence of CVD compared with whites), heredity, and aging. You certainly cannot change your race, bypass your ancestors' genes, or avoid getting older. With respect to aging, I always tell my patients: "If I had a pill to make you younger, I'd be taking it myself!"

Now the fact that some CVRF are unavoidable does not mean that they are not modifiable.

You may be genetically marked to have hypertension, high cholesterol levels, and diabetes, but that doesn't mean that you couldn't control them with excellent medical care.

SOME SUGGESTIONS ABOUT THE APPROACH TO CORRECT SOME CVRF

Smoking is the biggest preventable cause of premature mortality in the United States. Exposure to secondhand tobacco smoke is a significant risk for nonsmokers. Smoking causes the following deadly conditions:

- Cardiovascular disease: coronary and carotid cerebrovascular disease, abdominal aortic aneurysm
- Cancers: lung, oral (oral mucosa, tongue, laryngeal), esophagus, stomach, liver, pancreas, bladder, kidney, cervix, myeloid leukemia
- Respiratory disease: chronic obstructive pulmonary disease (COPD), pneumonia
- Reproductive effects: decreased fertility in women, complications of pregnancy (stillbirth, miscarriage, among others)

Interventions for Smoking Cessation

1- **Nicotine-based therapy:** transdermal patch, gum, nasal spray, inhaler, or lozenges
2- **Non-nicotine-based therapy:** non-nicotine-based therapy: drugs such as bupropion, varenicline, nortriptyline, clonidine

Sometimes a combination of the two methods improve results.

Hypertension. Beginning at 115/75 mmHg, the risk for CVD doubles with each 20 mmHg of systolic pressure elevation and 10 mmHg of diastolic pressure elevation.

The target systolic BP (blood pressure) is below 140 mmHg for most patients, below 130 mmHg in diabetic patients and patients with coronary artery disease, and below 120 mmHg in patients with nephropathy. In patients with congestive heart failure, the best BP is the lowest BP tolerated.

Serum lipids. Statin, nicotinic acid, and fibrates may all be used in persons with dyslipidemia (abnormalities of total cholesterol, HDL, LDL, and triglycerides), and in clinical trials these drugs have been shown to reduce cardiovascular events and slow or reverse angiographic progression of coronary atherosclerosis.

"Normal" serum lipid levels are reported as somewhat higher than those we mention below. For patients who have cardiovascular atherosclerotic disease and those who are at a high risk due to the presence of cardiovascular risk factors, some authorities recommend lipid levels as follows:

Total cholesterol: under 140 mg/dL
HDL "good cholesterol": over 50 mg/dL in men and over 55 mg/dL in women
LDL "bad cholesterol": under 70 mg/dL
Triglycerides: under 130 mg/dL

Other CVRF also need an aggressive, methodical, consistent, permanent approach to neutralize their dangerous tendency to damage arterial vessels in different areas of the human body: heart, brain, neck arteries, intestines, kidneys, penis, lower extremities. For example, diabetes control requires a glycohemoglobin under 7%, homocysteine levels may be lowered by folic acid; gum infections or other chronic infections (bronchitis, sinusitis) demand specific treatments.

CVRF are responsible for the high incidence of cardiovascular disease and many cases of rapid or sudden death. Your health care provider will help you with instructions and medications, but keep in mind that it is your behavioral changes and your own discipline to deal with them effectively that will prevent you from having a premature loss of life.

125—CIRCADIAN RHYTHM VARIATIONS

Circadian rhythms are the body's twenty-four-hour pattern of cyclical activity and have received attention by scientists for a number of years, most frequently with respect to the human sleep-wake cycle. Articles in the medical literature have reported the impact of circadian variations on blood pressure levels (highest in the early morning and then decline to a trough value after midnight and other cardiovascular events: anginal pains, myocardial infarctions, strokes, and sudden death, which appear to follow a similar pattern).

The observation of the circadian influences have led physicians to consider the prescription of cardiovascular drugs at special times, in an attempt to prevent uncomfortable and sometimes, dangerous complications.

Studies have shown the timing of the onset of coronary pains and acute myocardial infarctions peaked between the hours of 6:00 a.m. and noon. The Massachusetts death certificate study analyzed 2,203 death certificates of individuals who experienced out-of-hospital sudden cardiac deaths. The results were consistent with a circadian pattern with strong clustering occurring between 7:00 a.m. and 11:00 a.m. In fact, the risk of sudden cardiac death was approximately 70% between the hours of

7:00 a.m. and 9:00 a.m. compared with the average risk at other periods during the day.

HOW CIRCADIAN RHYTHMS MAY CONTRIBUTE TO ACUTE CARDIOVASCULAR EVENTS

At the time of awakening there is an increase in sympathetic system activity that translates into higher levels of circulating catecholamines (norepinephrine and epinephrine). This increases the blood pressure, the heart rate, and the constriction of coronary arteries.

At the same time, during the early morning hours, platelets tend to agglutinate more (they stick together), the viscosity (or "thickness") of the blood is more pronounced, and fibrinolytic activity, which normally helps to dissolve clots, suffers from laziness and that promotes clot formation inside the vessels.

If you have high blood pressure, discuss with your doctor the possibility of scheduling antihypertensive drugs in such a way that their major effect should be reserved for the early morning hours, after awakening.

Similar principles applied to cardiac medications, such as long-acting nitroglycerin, nitrate derivatives, calcium blockers, and beta-blockers.

126—COMMOTION CORDIS

Ironically, sometimes, a serious injury is survived, and a trivial one is not.

There's a difference between commotion of the heart and contusion of the heart. In the former, there's no heart damage. In the latter, there's tissue damage. Commotion cordis is a sudden disturbance of the cardiac rhythm that becomes chaotic following a blunt impact to the precordium, the area of the chest that overlies the heart. It usually happens in young people during sports activities. The condition is rare.

What causes it? Here are a few examples: the impact of a ball, a bat, a rubber or a plastic bullet, kicks, punches, pucks.

It is estimated that impact energies of at least 50 J are required to cause cardiac arrest when applied during the electrical vulnerable period of the cardiac cycle.

A hockey puck may hit a chest with an energy of 130 J, a karate punch may generate 450 J, and a heavyweight boxing champ may deliver a charge around 1,000 J.

Why does the heart stop beating in cases of commotion cordis?

Every heartbeat results from the pumping action of the left ventricle, the heart pump that ejects blood into the circulation. That is a mechanical action. What causes the contraction of the left ventricle is an electrical current generated by the heart itself. When this current reaches the heart muscle it "activates" it, and the heart contracts. The electrical system of the heart has sections that are invulnerable and others that are vulnerable. **Vulnerable means that if the heart is shaken by a commotion, it may generate a lethal rhythm called ventricular fibrillation. If the hit happens during the invulnerable period, this phenomenon will not take place.**

Ventricular fibrillation needs immediate action and conversion into a cardiac rhythm that is able to sustain life. There are many abnormal rhythms, but many of them produce an effective cardiac contraction. Ventricular fibrillation does not. Many abnormal rhythms allow us the time to deal with them effectively. If untreated, ventricular fibrillation is fatal.

Commotion cordis is a fulminant insult. Most victims don't make it. One important reason is that there's no one around who has the knowledge or the equipment (an automatic cardiac defibrillator) to do the job. This tragic end is responsible for the deaths of 2-3 very young individuals in the United States every year, and it is usually due to baseballs hitting the left anterior aspect of the thorax.

PREVENTION

The mandatory use of heavily padded vests in front of the thorax is generally sufficient to prevent high-energy impacts to the anterior left side of the chest (precordium).

Boxing is practiced with naked chests, cricket gears protect the legs but not the chest, and soccer . . . forget it, the only protection of the players is their own chest hair. The soccer ball weighs 450 g and may fly at a speed of 30 m/sec.

Parents should also supervise the kids playing in the backyard and adopt simple protective measures. These games can be as dangerous as professional sports activities.

127—DELAYED AND/OR INEFFECTIVE TREATMENT OF AN EMERGENCY DUE TO POOR ACCESS TO AN ADEQUATE MEDICAL FACILITY

To save a life in case of an emergency requires quick access to an adequate medical facility, trained personnel to provide effective treatment, and at times, advanced technology. Various actors and disciplines intervene in the process: police, rescue services, ambulance personnel, hospital staff, hospital technology.

In developed countries such as the United States, medical emergency services (MES) are often provided efficiently. But still, there are situations that end in tragedies.

Consider the case of small communities or those living in remote, isolated places. Carrying the patient by ambulance and/or other means to a medical center capable of dealing with the emergency is not an easy task. Patients are typically brought to an emergency department by private or by public transport (police ambulances, rescue services ambulances.

In some developing countries, coordination efforts to deal with such emergencies are even more difficult.

In developed and underdeveloped societies the management of emergencies is sometimes inadequate since some hospitals that receive the critically ill do not have the technical capability to provide a "state of the art" medical treatment in individual cases nor the capacity to deal with mass casualty situations.

Emergencies do occur in urban areas and in rural areas. EMS are mostly concentrated on urban areas. Wherever you live, **make sure you know how you could be taken fast to an emergency facility or a hospital that has the right equipment and the right professionals to save your life.**

Time for delivering appropriate emergency care is a crucial factor that impacts negatively on the outcome. Quality of medical care is essential too. In many hospitals there are deficiencies in the delivery of emergency treatment. Patients are not managed properly or have to wait long time before being treated. A patient's condition may deteriorate drastically in a very short period of time.

The management of emergency cases is a specialty field of its own that requires paramedical and medical personnel highly trained in this field. Currently, there are training programs for physicians, nurses, paramedical staff and **laymen.**

First-Aid skills can save lives. This training should also be provided for personnel that deals with public safety such as police, fire, security, traffic enforcers, school teachers, community volunteers, drivers, industrial workers, and also family members.

I advise you to do some research in your community on the availability of rescue teams, hospitals, quality of professional care, and technological advances, all of a which could give you the best chance of surviving an emergency situation such as a perforated appendix (peritonitis), hemorrhage, severe respiratory tract obstruction, a severe asthma attack, seizures, stroke, life-threatening cardiac arrhythmia, or an acute myocardial infarction, among many other potentially catastrophic conditions.

128—DIABETES

The first recognized episode of this disease may be the last.

Diabetes is a chronic disease and is capable of causing damage to the heart, kidneys, arterial system and other organs. The process takes years, and different individuals react differently to this disorder. Some sustain relatively mild complications. Others suffer plenty because of it. Diabetes may also cause acute complications that may be lethal in a few hours or days.

The disease has been around for several thousand years, and effective treatment was unavailable until insulin was extracted from pancreatic tissue in 1921. The estimated prevalence ranges from 3% to 10% of the population. Accelerated atherosclerosis produces 80% of all diabetic mortality, three-fourths of it owing to coronary disease.

Patients with type 1 diabetes have little or no insulin secretion, and the onset of the disease is usually abrupt with marked thirst (polydipsia), marked appetite (polyphagia), marked volumes of urine (polyuria), weight loss, and fatigue.

Patients with type 2 diabetes maintain some insulin secretory capability, but the body tissues offer resistance to the action of insulin. This results in elevated blood sugar levels (hyperglycemia).

DIABETIC KETOACIDOSIS

This is a life-threatening disorder resulting from poor control of diabetes and usually follows several days of increased thirst and urinary volumes. It can be a fulminant disease within a few hours. Those who carry an insulin pump must always remember that sometimes insulin pumps fail to function properly.

Diabetic ketoacidosis occurs in younger or older patients and in lean or obese individuals. The disorder is precipitated by emotional stress, severe acute cardiovascular events, excessive alcohol ingestion, trauma, infections, pregnancy. **At times, there's no recognizable precipitating cause.**

An abundance of ketone acids is characteristic of this disorder, and it may precipitate a comatose state. Therapy should be immediately started in a hospital's intensive care unit. Treatment is complex and must address cardiorespiratory, renal, cerebral, and electrolyte abnormalities. The precipitating cause of the diabetic ketoacidosis should be identified, if at all possible.

HYPERMOLAR NONKETOTIC COMA

This form of diabetic coma occurs less frequently than diabetic ketoacidosis. It is more common in the elderly diabetic individual and is rarely observed in younger patients. It is characterized by very high levels of blood glucose, usually greater than those accompanying diabetic ketoacidosis. Initial glucose concentration ranges from 600 to 2,400 mg/dL. Death is usually the result of increased coagulability of the blood (platelets abnormalities) and thrombosis (clot formation in brain and coronary arteries).

HYPOGLYCEMIC COMA

Hypoglycemia should always be considered in any patient brought to the emergency room in coma.

In known diabetic patients on insulin or oral hypoglycemic agents, hypoglycemia is a likely cause of coma. The presence of or a recent history of seizures in elderly patients should raise the suspicion of hypoglycemic coma.

Blood glucose levels under 50 mg/dL should be considered to be due to hypoglycemia coma until proven otherwise. Therapy with 50% dextrose solution should be initiated at once.

129—DISSEMINATED INTRAVASCULAR COAGULATION PLUS KIDNEY FAILURE

This is a very dramatic development that clearly represents a nightmare for the patient and for the treating physicians as well. There are various degrees of severity, but when disseminated, intravascular coagulation (DIC) means business (and it always does). It follows a quick and destructive course of catastrophic proportions.

This disorder is usually seen in patients suffering from severe sepsis (abundance of bacteria in the bloodstream), retained placentas, or a dead fetus. The patient develops a bleeding disorder and may bleed from the nose, the rectum, the urine, the brain. Actually, the bleeding may happen in any organ of the human body. Even the venous punctures ooze blood that characteristically cannot be stopped by pressing the little needle opening with a sponge. And the oozing continues for days.

What happens in the patient's blood is as follows: Thrombin is a substance that circulates in the blood and increases its levels significantly in DIC. Its usual role is to activate fibrinogen and convert it into fibrin. Since the amount of thrombin is excessive, the blood tends to coagulate inside the veins and arteries. At the same time, this disease produces factors that lower the number of platelets, and this causes hemorrhages. Renal failure is a common complication and makes a bad situation worse.

Treatment of DIC requires intensive therapy with antibiotics to fight sepsis, removal of the retained placenta, or delivery of the dead fetus, all of it, on emergency basis.

130—DROWNING

Sometimes it's an accident; sometimes, it's neglect.

This death occurs by suffocation when excessive amount of water in the lungs prevent the absorption of oxygen from the air. This causes hypoxia (decreased oxygen content in tissues) and the accumulation of toxic acids in the blood (acidosis). Both of these lead to a cardiac arrest.

Drowning is common. In the United States there are 6,500 episodes per year or about 1 per 50,000 of population. It is the fifth cause of accidental death in the country. Victims are usually teenagers. Studies indicate that 10% of children under five have experienced a situation with a high risk of drowning.

CAUSES OF DROWNING

- 44% swimming
- 17% boating
- 14% uncertain
- 10% scuba diving
- 7% car accidents

OCCURENCES OF DROWNING

90% in rivers, lakes, and pools
10% in seawater

RISK FACTORS

- Males are more likely to drown than females
- Failure to wear protective equipment when boating
- Poor supervision of children under five
- Entrapment by clothing or equipment
- Drugs and alcohol
- Injury, fatigue, cold water temperature
- Heart attack, severe cardiac arrhythmia, stroke, or seizure while in the water deep-breath-hold dive blackout
- Murder

Children have drowned in buckets, baths, and toilets.

MECHANISM OF DEATH IN DROWNING

A person in danger of drowning holds his/her breath (apnea). During the process, oxygen in the blood decreases, and carbon dioxide increases. The latter leads to a stronger breathing reflex, and when it reaches a breaking point, the victim can no longer hold his or her breath. There's a laryngeal spasm or constriction that acts as a defensive mechanism trying to avoid passage of water into the lungs. This is important because artificial respiration is much more effective when water has not entered the lungs.

A continued lack of oxygen in the brain will lead to unconsciousness. The brain dies after six minutes without oxygen, but cold water will somewhat protect the brain. The same lack of oxygen in the body will cause a cardiac arrest.

THE RESCUE EFFORT

- Many pools and bathing areas have lifeguards, a pool safety camera system, or computer-aided drowning detection
- Bystanders are important and should call for help immediately
- A lifeguard is to be called fast
- No person should attempt a rescue that is beyond his or her capacity
- If you're trying to rescue a drowning victim, bring the victim's mouth and nose above the water surface and remove the victim from the water
- Some victims panic and try to cling to the rescuer submerging him or her in the process. In such cases, try to twist the victim's arm on the back to restrict movement
- If the victim pushes you, the rescuer, underwater, dive downward to escape the victim. Ensure your own safety
- In water, CPR is ineffective. If possible, bring the victim to a stable ground as quickly as possible and start CPR, and ask another person to call rescue
- The Heimlich maneuver, so useful in other cases of upper airway obstruction by a solid object, should not be applied when suffocation is due to airway obstruction by fluids. This maneuver in drowning victims may induce vomiting, which is aspirated, making matters worse
- Drowning victim resuscitation efforts should be made even to victims who were submerged for a long time. Children in particular have a

good chance of survival when they have been in water up to 3 or 10 minutes in cold water (10-15 °C or 50-60 °F). Submersion in cold water slows the metabolism and the need for oxygen dramatically. There have been miraculous recoveries with victims who have been immersed for long periods of time. In one case, a child named Michelle Frank survived after being submerged for 70 minutes, and in another, an eighteen-year-old male survived 38 minutes under the water

PREVENTION

- Learn to swim, and do it under supervision
- If you swim at the sea, do it close to the beach. Don't go too far
- Swim in areas where there's a lifeguard
- Wear a lifejacket with water sports such as sailing, surfing, or canoeing
- Pay attention to weather conditions, tides, and water currents
- Watch children closely
- Don't swim alone
- Never swim if you consumed alcohol or drugs
- Know your limitations and have reverence and respect for them
- Never dive into the water unless you clearly see the bottom or know its depth

When I was a teenager I went for a swimming in the sea up to about 300 feet from the beach and enjoyed playing with huge waves. One time, I almost had lunch with a shark. (Please see section 173). At that age, I thought that what I was doing was adventurous and exciting. Today, I define it as immaturity and stupidity.

131—ELECTROCUTION

In my professional practice as a cardiologist, on numerous occasions, I had to apply an electrical current over the thorax of people who had a cardiac arrhythmia. This technique is called cardioversion. Sometimes, it is done in patients who feel comfortable (elective cardioversion) or under more dramatic circumstances, when the arrhythmia is causing a state of heart failure, shock, acute chest pain or shortness of breath, low blood pressure (hypotension), or severe palpitations. In such cases, the procedure is carried out on emergency basis.

An electrical current applied to the chest of a normal person may cause a cardiac arrest. The same current applied to the chest to convert an arrhythmia may be lifesaving.

When I was a medical resident, I applied the pad electrodes to a patient's chest to convert an arrhythmia, and accidentally, I barely touched the bed with my thighs. The shock reached me and shook my entire body me badly. It was a terrible sensation! And the voltage I received was low (30 v)!

Electrocution is a major cause of injury and death in both the industrial and home environment. Most electrocution injuries occur at voltages above 50 volts AC or 100 volts DC. A deadly voltage, however, can be much lower.

The electrocution voltage for humans is very low: for adults it is about 10 milliamps and for small children, 5 milliamps.

Most industrial electrocution and electrical injuries are caused by either code violations or a defective product or human error and are preventable.

There are many electrical accidents in homes that cause over 4,000 cases per year seen at emergency departments. The National Institutes of Health estimates that there are 1,000 deaths annually in the United States caused by electric shock.

Prolonged exposure to currents greater than 18 milliamps across the chest causes the diaphragm to contract, which prevents breathing and causes suffocation.

Once electricity makes contact with the human body, this may go into a cardiac arrest or affect muscles, nerves, and tissues that can be damaged due to the current. Sometimes, burns result.

Microshock electrocution may be caused by failures in the hospital electrical system or by electrical equipment that comes into contact with the patient. These deficiencies can be found if properly tested by the appropriate equipment.

The severity of the injuries depends on the intensity of the voltage, the person's state of health, how the current has traveled through the victim's body, and how quickly medical assistance is provided.

Electrocution may or may not leave physical evidence of the injury. The presence of burns depends upon the current density at the point of entrance of the current.

ELECTROCUTION IN THE HOME ENVIRONMENT

Extension cords

These can cause electrical burns and shock. Cords that have exposed wires should never be used. Kids and pets tend to chew them. Even an intact extension cord may be dangerous. In one case, a fifteen-month-old girl put an extension cord in her mouth and suffered electrical burns that required surgery.

How to avoid trouble

- Purchase extension cords that have been subjected to strict testing and safety standards
- Keep extension cords out of reach of children and pets
- Inspect them regularly for signs of wear and tear
- Replace cords that are cracked
- Pull the plug, not the cord when disconnecting it from the socket
- Only use extension cords when they are absolutely necessary

Electrical outlets

- Cover outlets so children cannot insert their fingers or objects into them

Electric appliances

Even touching an electric appliance like a hair dryer with wet hands can cause a shock.

Safety tips

- Don't use electrical appliances near water or while touching faucets or water pipes
- Don't use appliances that have worn plugs or cracked wires
- Don't try to fix an electrical appliance on your own
- Unplug appliances you are not using

Swimming pools, hot tubs, spas

Risks come from the following:

- Faulty underwater lighting
- Aging electrical wiring
- Sump pumps
- Electrical appliances and extension cords that fall into the water

The risks are higher when lightning and circuits aren't protected by ground fault circuit interrupters (GFCIs). This is a great protection against electrocution.

Power Lines

High voltage overhead power lines can pose a risk to people on ladders or other lifts.

Never place a ladder, antenna, or anything else near a power line. Consumers who come in contact with an overhead power line may not survive to tell the story. Wires from a downed power line may kill instantly. **Be careful after the storm.** Don't step on it! Don't touch it!

People have also been electrocuted in a car accident when the car hit an electrical pole and the live wires touched the car.

Lightning: see section 149

132—EMOTIONAL REACTIONS—PSYCHOLOGICAL DISORDERS

There are many anecdotal as well as medically documented cases of persons who died suddenly following a severe emotional reaction. Intense fear, "being scared to death," or bouts of intense anger are known to produce lethal arrhythmias.

People who suffer from depression and hopelessness are more likely than others to suffer heart attacks and sudden cardiac death. They are also more likely to develop conditions that increase heart risk, such as obesity, diabetes, and hypertension.

An emotional impact, such as the death of a spouse, posttraumatic stress disorder, or even a substantial financial loss increase the risk of myocardial infarctions and sudden death.

I once admitted a patient to the hospital with acute chest pains hours after he had learned of a loss of 300,000 dollars at the stock market. A few hours following hospitalization, he had a cardiac arrest and could not be resuscitated.

Acute fear may end in disaster too. At 4:31 a.m., on January 17, 1994, a violent earthquake near Northridge, California, suddenly awakened millions of people in Los Angeles. The earthquake caused victims by physical damage, but there was a large number of deaths due to cardiovascular disease because of the intense fright caused by the natural disaster.

Socioeconomic factors, intense grief, marital discrepancies, the breakup of a significant relationship, a deeply disappointing and humiliating experience, the discovery of a life-threatening illness or disabling condition, the loss of a job and no income in the household, or a big unexpected noise can also precipitate sudden cardiac death.

Death due to emotional stress results from the effects of excessive adrenaline on the heart by causing constriction of coronary arteries and myocardial infarctions and fatal arrhythmias.

133—EUTHANASIA

Euthanasia is a medically assisted death. For many centuries it's been a subject of debate. It essentially consists of a practice to help a person who suffers a torment with pain or just has a few months to live to end her/his life.

Euthanasia always had devoted advocates and resolute enemies. There seems to be nothing in between these two extremes. People love it or hate it. Those who are in favor or this "aid in dying" believe it is merciful. Those who are against it consider it a form of murder.

Despite these diametrically opposite points of view, some compromise has been acceptable by some societies, some countries, and some religions.

Euthanasia may be carried out with consent, voluntary euthanasia, or without consent, involuntary euthanasia. This procedure, without consent, would apply to people who are incapable of making a decision, and this is left to a proxy. As you can imagine, this option is extraordinarily controversial. For many, it equals to murder.

Euthanasia may be conducted in the following ways:

* *Passive*. It withholds some treatments (antibiotics, surgery) or increases the doses and frequency of morphine injections knowing that this may shorten life. This is the most accepted form of euthanasia, and it's commonly practiced in most hospitals
* *Nonaggressive*. It withdraws life support. This alternative is more controversial
* *Aggressive*. This uses lethal substances that kill the person. This is the most controversial form of euthanasia

Hippocrates mentions in his Hippocratic oath: "To please no one will I prescribe a deadly drug nor give advice which may cause his death." This declaration goes back to 400-300 years BC. But that was his personal opinion. Ancient Greeks and Romans had a different perspective and did not believe that life needed to be preserved at any cost. They were consequently tolerant of suicide in cases where no relief could be offered to the dying.

In the Middle Ages, English common law made suicide a criminal act in England. Assisting another to kill themselves remains illegal in that country. The first antieuthanasia law in the United States was passed in the State of New York in 1828, and other states followed suit. Over the years in England and the United States, there were organized groups that promoted aggressive euthanasia methods, but legislation was not approved.

In 1990, Dr. Jack Kevorkian, a Michigan physician, almost made a sport of killing people by assisting them to commit suicide. He claimed to have assisted at least 130 patients to die. A Michigan jury convicted him in 1999 for second-degree murder to a ten-to-twenty-five-year prison sentence but only served eight years due to failing health. He was released on June 1, 2007.

Dr. Kevorkian assisted people to die by attaching the individual to a device that he had made. The person pushed a button, and drugs or chemicals were released into the individual's venous system that would end his or her own life. He called it a Thanatron (death machine). Other people were assisted by a different device, which employed a gas mask that delivered carbon monoxide, and he called it Mercitrhon (mercy machine). In 1990, the Supreme Court approved the use of nonaggressive euthanasia (IV fluids restrictions, withdrawal of antibiotics, artificial respiration methods, surgery).

One more recent case was that of Terri Schiavo, a Floridian who vegetated since 1990 and had her feeding tube removed in 2005. Her husband won the right to take her off life support. The husband claimed that Terri would have never wanted that kind of survival but had left no living will. Her family disagreed and wanted to keep the feeding tube to the end, but Mr. Schiavo's argument prevailed.

EUTHANASIA AND RELIGION

Jewish and Protestant medical ethics have become divided on euthanasia since the 1970s. Orthodox Jews oppose voluntary euthanasia although there's some flexibility for voluntary passive euthanasia. Conservative and Reform Judaism have shown increasing support for certain methods of passive euthanasia.

Roman Catholics tend to strongly oppose active euthanasia, but the Church has left some room for limited forms of passive euthanasia "when inevitable death is imminent." It was permitted to take the decision to refuse forms of treatment that would secure a burdensome prolongation of life, as long as the normal care due to a sick person is not interrupted.

Islam forbids all forms of suicide and any action that may help another to kill themselves. If, however, an individual is suffering from an incurable illness, it is permissible for him/her to refuse medication, resuscitation, dialysis for renal failure, or chemotherapy for cancer.

Buddhism prohibits any form of euthanasia. Instead of trying to ease the individual's transition to death, it focuses on easing his or her insight into suffering and its end.

During many years of medical practice, I had to deal with terminally ill patients who suffered intolerable pain. One of the hospitals I was associated with for a period of twenty-five years was a Catholic institution. Rules and ethical standards were strict. Special hospital committees supervised cases of dying patients and analyzed the procedures used by the doctors in the handling of such cases. I've always felt that if, as a doctor, I was unable to help a patient to survive, at least, I should do whatever was in my power to help him or her to die. I did that on numerous occasions and never had a problem with the hospital's rules and regulations. Whenever possible, I discussed the situation with the patient's family and at times with the priest on duty. The chosen method was passive euthanasia and often involved the use of morphine every 4-6 hours around the clock. This allowed patients to avoid pain and discomforts, and usually the demise occurred in a few days. Invariably, the patient's relatives provided me with expressions of gratitude for acting that way.

134—EXERCISE

Overall, physical activity decreases cardiovascular disease risk, but there's also a risk of sudden death associated with physical exercise. Estimates about the incidence of this phenomenon vary. In a study of high school and college athletes, the absolute exercise-related death rate was 1 per 133,000 men and 1 per 769,000 women per year. These estimates included all sports-related nontraumatic deaths.

In Seattle, Washington, USA, the annual incidence of exercise-related cardiac arrests among previously healthy adults was 1 for every 18,000.

CAUSES OF SUDDEN DEATH DURING EXERCISE

Age is an important factor to predict the possible cause of a sudden death during exercise. Most young athletes die of non-atherosclerotic heart disease. This means that disease of the coronary arteries is generally not the cause of death.

Hypertrophic cardiomyopathy, a congenital disease characterized by a thick heart muscle that blocks the exit of blood from the left ventricle, is the predominant cause of death in young athletes occurring in up to 50% of all cases.

Those older than thirty-five years typically die of coronary atherosclerosis. In this group, coronary atherosclerosis is responsible for about 80% of sudden deaths. Only 50% of them have some warning symptoms.

HOW EXERCISE PROVOKES AN ACUTE CORONARY FATAL EVENT

Several hypotheses have been postulated to explain how exercise might provoke acute coronary events.

- Acute spasm of a coronary artery
- Rupture of an atherosclerotic plaque. Physical exertion increases the pressure inside the coronary arteries, thereby increasing shear forces that contribute to plaque rupture. Exercise provokes exaggerated changes in cardiac dimensions, which may stimulate plaque disintegration. **Remember: A ruptured atherosclerotic plaque means clot formation, and clot formation means obstruction of the coronary artery and an acute myocardial infarction**

OTHER LESS FREQUENT CAUSES OF SUDDEN CARDIAC DEATH DURING EXERCISE (LESS THAN 5% OF SUDDEN CARDIAC DEATH)

- Arrhythmogenic right ventricular dysplasia
- Left ventricular hypertrophy of unknown cause
- Dilated cardiomyopathy due to various causes
- Myocarditis
- Long QT syndrome
- Drug abuse (cocaine is always a prime suspect)
- Aortic stenosis
- Mitral valve prolapse
- Rupture of an aortic aneurysm (Marfan's syndrome)
- Wolf-Parkinson-White (WPW) syndrome
- Kawasaki disease
- Sarcoidosis
- Sickle cell trait
- Commotion cordis

PREVENTION

Several attempts have been made to identify high-risk athletes, hoping that this will prevent sudden cardiac deaths. Echocardiograms are negative in thousands of cases. So it turned out to be impractical to do them. Mitral valve prolapse is not itself a contraindication to exercise. It is therefore not recommended to do routine echocardiographic screening in young athletes.

In older athletes, it's a different story. The American College of Sports Medicine recommends routine use of exercise testing to screen high-risk individuals before vigorous exercise.

It is recommended that young athletes undergo a cardiovascular examination including, of course, a carefully taken medical history. Those who present abnormalities should have further evaluation.

135—EXERCISE STRESS TESTING

Exercise test is regularly done in medical practice using the treadmill with the purpose of discovering coronary artery disease, also to assess the capacity to exercise or quantify the degree of disability, estimate prognosis, and monitor patients with chronic obstructive pulmonary disease.

The test is generally safe although it is estimated that approximately 1 person dies and 5 have nonfatal complications per 10,000 cases.

The test must be carried out with available emergency equipment that is safe and accurate. There are contraindications for stress testing, and it is very important to keep them in mind.

Contraindications

- Acute myocardial infarction (within two days)
- Unstable angina
- Severe aortic stenosis
- Congestive heart failure
- Acute myocarditis
- Acute pericarditis
- Acute aortic dissection
- A large thoracic or abdominal aortic aneurysm
- Severe hypertension
- Severe tachycardia or bradycardia
- Advanced heart block
- Severe electrolyte abnormalities
- Severe obstructive cardiomyopathy
- Mental or physical impairment that does not allow adequate treadmill performance

Indications to Terminate a Treadmill Stress Test

- A drop in systolic blood pressure during exercise
- Chest pain, significant shortness of breath, or excessive fatigue
- Turning pale and blue of the patient and having cold skin
- Patient requesting to stop the test
- Occurrence of serious arrhythmias
- Technical difficulties during the test that make adequate monitoring difficult
- Marked development of electrocardiographic abnormalities

136—GASTROINTESTINAL BLEEDING

Hematemesis is defined as the vomiting of blood, and *melena* is defined as the passage of stools of black color and tarry appearance due to altered blood. These occur because of diseases of the esophagus, stomach, and duodenum. Melena may also occur with bleeding from the small bowel and even the ascending colon.

A blood loss of 500 mL may not cause a significant problem in young patients, but the elderly is particularly vulnerable. The same susceptibility occurs in patients who are already anemic when the episode of bleeding strikes.

Causes of upper gastrointestinal bleeding include peptic ulcer disease, gastritis, endoscopy (introduction of an instrument in the esophagus and stomach for diagnostic purposes), esophageal varices resulting from liver disease. Liver scarring impairs the venous circulation and creates a pressure inside the venous system that is transmitted to the esophagus. This happens in alcoholic cirrhotic livers or those livers scarred by hepatitis.

Colonic diverticuli, localized packets, usually multiple, can also bleed massively. The blood passed per rectum, though, will be red, not black.

All patients who develop acute gastrointestinal bleeding need urgent assessment and admission to the hospital. Those who present with hematemesis tend to have more severe bleeding than those who present with melena alone. Hospital mortality is approximately 10%, and prime victims are elderly patients who suffer from cardiovascular, respiratory, and cerebrovascular disease. Many patients' bleeding is associated with the use of anti-inflammatory drugs.

137—GUILLAIN-BARRE SYNDROME

I've seen patients with this disease dying in a few days with respiratory failure. It is an acute polyneuropathy. It begins with paralysis of the lower extremities, and then the process extends to the upper limbs. Respiratory assistance with a ventilator is necessary in about 30% of cases. Nowadays, the prognosis is generally good, and the mortality rate is 3-4%. That was not the case when I saw patients dying with a severe and fulminant form of Guillain-Barre in the 1960s. The origin of this malady is unknown: a virus or an immune-mediated mechanism seems to be the most likely cause.

138—HEMOLYTIC ANEMIA

Hemolysis means blood's red cells destruction. The phenomenon has multiple causes. Some are hereditary. Examples are the following: hereditary spherocytosis is the most common of its kind and affects individuals of Northern European extraction. When severe, it may be life threatening. Sickle cell anemia occasionally turns nasty, and the crisis it leads to may be fatal. Others are provoked by autoimmune disorders; drugs such as pyridium, dapsone and other sulfones, chemicals. Even mechanical prosthetic cardiac valves sometimes destroy red blood cells.

Hemolytic anemias are at times severe, and blood transfusions improve the patient's status and stabilize the situation. But there are certain hemolytic anemias that are particularly dangerous. Certain forms of malaria can be malignant. The parasites enter the red cells and break them.

There is an intracellular organism called *Babesia microti* that causes babesion, an infection that is endemic to coastal New England and is transmitted by ticks. Some bacteria are extremely dangerous and when they cause sepsis and are not treated emergently with antibiotics, they can be fatal. Two of the most notorious examples are given by *Bartonella baciliformis*, a bacterium transmitted by the sand fly (bartonellosis or Oroya fever) and the massive hemolysis provoked by the *Clostridium perfringens*.

139—HYPERCALCEMIA

This is an abnormal elevation of serum calcium levels.

Calcium plays an important role in muscular contraction, nerve conduction, blood coagulation, electrolyte regulation, and hormone release. Calcium, in turn, is tightly regulated by a series of hormones that affect calcium mobilization from the bone and gastrointestinal tract and its excretion through the kidneys.

A normal total serum calcium level is 8-10 mg/dL, and hypercalcemia exists when its level is greater than 10.5 mL/dL. According to the serum calcium levels, hypercalcemia can be the following:

Calcium serum levels
Mild: 10.5-11.9 mg/dL
Moderate: 12-13.9 mg/dL
Severe (also called hypercalcemic crisis): 14-16 mg/dL

Calcium is regulated by the parathyroid hormone, calcitonin, and vitamin D.

Hypercalcemia mainly affects the central nervous system and the kidneys. It can cause fatigue, depression, personality changes, and confusion. **With very high levels, somnolence, coma, and death may ensue.**

Calcium excess in the circulating blood is excreted through the kidneys, and stones are formed (nephrolithiasis). Calcium also causes constriction of the renal arteries and that leads to **hypertension. In the heart, hypercalcemia may affect the conducting (or electrical) system and cause cardiac arrhythmias.**

Significance of Hypercalcemia

Hypercalcemia due to excess of parathyroid hormone is usually mild and chronic.

Hypercalcemia caused by a malignant tumor tends to be much more serious. Some malignant tumors have the capacity to produce a factor that acts similarly to the parathyroid hormone. This hormone increases the calcium serum levels. Malignancies may also produce hypercalcemia due to destructive bone action from metastatic lesions (metastasis means that a cancerous tumor of a certain organ extended to the bones). When it's severe, hypercalcemia due to malignancies may lead to death.

Other Causes of Hypercalcemia

- Physical immobilization
- Thiazide diuretics
- Hyperthyroidism
- Vitamin D
- Hyperparathyroidism (increased production of parathyroid hormone by the parathyroid gland)
- Milk-Alkaline syndrome (due to excessive calcium carbonate consumption to treat osteoporosis, dyspepsia, or hyperphosphatemia [high serum levels of phosphorus]) in patients with severe renal failure

I once interviewed a couple at my office. He was sixty-four; she was twenty-three. He had gold chains in his neck, and more gold in his wrists and hands. He dressed like a teenager and complained of easy fatigability, easy irritability, and a tendency to fall asleep at daytime. Her girlfriend had exactly similar complaints. I asked them if they had been taking vitamin D. She said that he'd been consuming seventy multivitamins tablets a day for quite a while. Since she did not want him to be sensitive about his age and his desire to look and act as a young person, she also took seventy multivitamins tablets a day. Their serum calcium was around 13.8 mg/ dL. I urged both of them to stop taking vitamins. Calcium levels returned to normal in a few days.

These two cases reflected vitamin D intoxication.

TREATMENT

Treatment for hypercalcemia aims both at lowering of serum calcium concentration and doing whatever is possible to eliminate or decrease the underlying disease.

The basic treatment of hypercalcemia begins with intravenous saline solution administration to produce volume expansion and increased excretion of urinary calcium. Then, specific therapy must deal with the specific cause of this disorder.

140—HYPERKALEMIA

Hyperkalemia is an elevated blood level of electrolyte potassium. Severe serum potassium elevation represents a medical emergency because it may produce fatal arrhythmias.

The trouble with hyperkalemia is that it is often undetected until a serious complication occurs, namely, a serious cardiac rhythm disturbance or sudden death.

Symptoms of hyperkalemia are not specific. Weakness, palpitations, muscular weakness may be present.

CAUSES

- Renal insufficiency
- Medications that reduce the urinary excretion of potassium
    * ACE inhibitors and angiotensin receptor blockers
    * Certain diuretics (amiloride, spironolactone)
    * Ibuprofen, naproxen, celecoxib
    * Trimethoprim (antibiotic)
    * Pentamidine (antiparasitic drug)
    * Ciclosporin and tacrolimus (immunosuppressants)
- Some hormonal deficiencies
    * Addison's disease (adrenal gland insufficiency)
    * Aldosterone deficiency, sometimes it is due to the effect of a blood thinner (heparin)
- Gordon's syndrome ("familial hypertension with hyperkalemia), a rare genetic disorder
- Cellular destruction
    * Burns that cause rapid muscular destruction (rhabdomyolysis)
    * Massive blood transfusion or massive hemolysis (destruction of red blood cells)
    * Shifts in transport of potassium caused by acidosis, low insulin levels, beta-blockers, digitalis overdose
    * Excessive intake
    * Overdose by tablets or intravenous administration
- Lethal injection

Hyperkalemia is used as part of the **legal execution process by lethal injection**, potassium chloride being the third and last of the three drugs administered to cause death, after sodium thiopental has rendered the individual unconscious. Then, pancuronium bromide is added to cause respiratory collapse.

CAUTION ABOUT FALSELY ELEVATED SERUM POTASSIUM LEVELS

This may occur during venipuncture when excessive vacuum of the blood drawn or by a syringe that has a very small needle, excessive tourniquet time, or fist clenching during blood extraction, or a delay in processing the blood specimen.

Electrocardiogram shows typical changes according to the severity of hyperkalemia.

TREATMENT

Serum potassium levels that exceed 6.5 mmol/L must be considered a medical emergency and must be lowered as soon as possible. Calcium gluconate at 10%, insulin plus dextrose at 50%, sodium bicarbonate and other medications are available to deal with this condition. When the potassium levels are dangerously high and do not respond to drugs, dialysis must be considered.

141—HYPERTHERMIA

This condition develops acutely when the body produces or absorbs more heat than it can dissipate. It is usually due to excessive heat exposure. The body mechanisms that normally regulate the heat are overwhelmed, and the temperature climbs up like a crazy horse. It is a medical emergency.

Normal body temperature is from 36 to 37 °C (97-98 °F). Temperatures above 40 °C (104 °F) create a life-threatening situation. At 41 °C (106 °F) brain death begins, and at 45 °C (113 °F), death is imminent. Above 50 °C (122 °F), death occurs immediately.

Heat exhaustion or heat prostration presents with nausea or vomiting, mental confusion, muscular cramps, and excessive sweating. When the temperature rises to 39-40 °C range (103-104 °F), heat exhaustion progresses to **heat stroke**. Perspiration helps at the beginning of the process because it draws heat from the body. Trouble is that when the body becomes dehydrated and there's no more sweating, the body temperature begins its trip to the sky. The victim is confused, may have a headache, and the blood pressure drops due to dehydration. This causes dizziness or fainting. The heart rate increases and respiration gets agitated. Trembling and chills follow. Children often have convulsions. When the heat stroke advances even further, there is temporary blindness; the body functions collapse, and coma ensues.

FIRST AID

- Heat stroke is an emergency that requires immediate hospitalization
- The temperature must be lowered fast. The victim needs to be moved to a cooler area such as corridor or the shade, his/her clothes removed and placed in cool water or wrapped in a cool wet towel. A fan, ice, and very cold water are useful, but the body temperature must be monitored closely to avoid hypothermia
- If the person is to be immersed in a bathtub of cold water, four to five people are necessary, and the head should be kept above water
- Hydration is essential. Water and sports drinks should be used
- Alcohol and caffeine should be avoided. These act as diuretics and aggravate dehydration
- Alcohol rubs are hazardous: these also cause further dehydration
- Place the victim in the recovery position (see index) to keep the airway open

PREVENTION

Don't leave children in enclosed spaces such as cars. In hot weather people need to drink lots of fluid to compensate for the profuse perspiration.

WHO ARE THE LIKELY VICTIMS OF HEAT STROKE

- The poor
- The elderly
- Urban dwellers
- Young children
- Patients with physical or mental illnesses
- Substance users and abusers
- Those who engage in intense physical activities under difficult conditions and hot weather

142—HYPOCALCEMIA

This is a lower than normal level of serum calcium, and it was one of my first exposures to medical practice. I was in the last year of my medical career and ready for MD graduation. I was working at the emergency room of a hospital in the Greater Buenos Aires area, Argentina, when a father rushed into the ER crying and carrying his nine-year-old son who was unconscious and unresponsive. At the moment, I had no doctor to consult. I was alone in the ER with a couple of nurses. I was the only one who could take care of that emergency immediately. The child looked more dead than alive. I checked his BP, and when the cuff around his arm was tightened, it caused a spasm of his hand called carpal spasm, which I recognized from the previous reading of an endocrinologist textbook and which had shown a photo with that sign, characteristic of hypocalcemia. I instantly injected calcium gluconate intravenously, and to my total surprise and the father's exhilarating happiness, the kid opened his eyes, moved all of the extremities well. His blood pressure and pulse became detectable. He saw his father and asked him: "Dad, what happened to me?"

The father hugged me and kissed me and was crying uncontrollably. The child had severe hypocalcemia. He was transferred to a specialized facility for an in-depth search of the cause of his hypocalcemia.

General Concepts on Calcium

Calcium is critically important for normal cell function, nerve transmission, bone structure, blood coagulation, among other functions. If hypocalcemia, which is lower serum levels of calcium, is not discovered on time and happens to be severe, it may lead to death.

WHAT SEVERE HYPOCALCEMIA DOES

- Severe hypocalcemia may cause cardiovascular collapse, a very low blood pressure (hypotension), which does not easily respond to injection of fluids or drugs to raise it
- At times, the disease that caused hypocalcemia, may be the real threat, more so than hypocalcemia itself
- Serious cardiac arrhythmias, shortness of breath and bronchospasm, tingling sensations, fainting, heart failure, angina and seizures may occur
- **Death is rare, but it has happened.**

CAUSES

There are numerous causes of hypocalcemia. I'll mention those who are mostly seen during emergent situations.

A low level of albumin in the blood, hypoalbuminemia, is the most frequent cause of hypocalcemia. Hypoalbuminemia occurs in cirrhosis, nephrosis, burns, malnutrition, chronic illness, sepsis. Low calcium in the blood associated with low serum albumin needs a special corrective formula to determine the correct calcium levels.

- Acute pancreatitis
- Rhabdomyolysis or extensive muscular damage
- Toxic shock
- Sepsis
- Malignancies (some cause hypercalcemia and some produce hypocalcemia)
- Liver or kidney failure
- Poisoning with ingestion of hydrofluoric acid
- High citrate states, e.g., massive blood transfusions
- Severe vitamin D deficiency

MEDICATIONS THAT CAN PRODUCE HYPOCALCEMIA

- Proton pump inhibitors reduce gastric production and that results in reduced calcium absorption
- Phenytoin
- Phenobarbital
- Fluoride
- Estrogens
- Alcohol
- Others

DIAGNOSIS

A calcium level less than 8.5 mg/dL is considered hypocalcemia. PTH levels, kidney and liver functions tests, serum albumin levels, magnesium, phosphorus, and other electrolytes are all essential.

Mild hypocalcemia is not an emergency and needs workup to disclose its possible cause. Severe hypocalcemia needs observation and treatment in an intensive care unit. Supportive care is provided:

oxygen, intravenous fluids, treatment of arrhythmias and seizures. The magic medication is calcium gluconate in injections given in a five—to ten-minute period.

Hypocalcemia may be a complex disorder. It may require the intervention of the internist, endocrinologist, oncologist, nephrologist, intensivist, surgeon, and toxicologist.

The **prognosis and outlook** of hypocalcemia depends upon its cause, but it's generally good.

143—HYPOGLYCEMIA

This condition occurs when the blood sugar levels are lower than normal. It is a frequent problem in patients with diabetes who are taking hypoglycemic drugs, and the problem is generally corrected by the immediate consumption of sugar or something that contains it.

Two cases of severe hypoglycemia I had to deal with and that I could never forget were those of an attorney who had an insulinoma (a pancreatic tumor that produces large amounts of insulin) and an elderly female who committed suicide by swallowing many tablets of an oral medication she was taking for diabetes. (Please see section on suicide.)

A patient with insulinoma was a very pleasant gentleman who became psychotic and violent when his blood sugars dropped to critically low levels. Some of these attacks occurred in the bathroom. He was perspiring profusely and screaming all kinds of profanities. I managed to give him intravenous injection of concentrated dextrose. Almost immediately, he calmed down and asked me in the sweetest possible way: "Where am I? What happened to me?"

Hypoglycemia may result from medications, hormone deficiencies, or tumors.

Diabetic patients more often go into coma because of hypoglycemia rather than high blood levels of glucose.

Glucose is a form of sugar, and it is a very important fuel for our bodies. Carbohydrates are the main food sources of glucose. Potatoes, rice, breads, tortillas, ice cream, cereal, milk, fruit, and all sweets contain plenty of glucose.

SYMPTOMS

- Acute anxiety
- Weakness
- Sleepiness
- Confusion
- Slurred speech
- Perspiration
- Shakiness
- Dizziness

All of the above are noted while you are awake. Hypoglycemia may occur during the sleep.

- You might have nightmares
- Find your bed sheets or pajamas wet from excessive perspiration
- Feel tired, irritable, or confused when you wake up

People who are taking medications for diabetes may develop hypoglycemia if

- they take excessive doses of insulin or an oral hypoglycemic agent meals or snacks are delayed, skipped, or too small;
- they exercise in excess; have drank alcohol excessively

PREVENTION

- Be careful about the way you take oral medications for diabetes or insulin. Only take the recommended doses and at the right time
- Have a meal plan prepared by a nutritionist or endocrinologist and that you find adequate according to your personal taste
- Get advice from your doctor about snacks
- Be careful with alcohol. It can cause hypoglycemia, particularly if it is drunk on an empty stomach. If you drink alcohol, have a snack or a meal at the same time. Binge drinking is the worse kind. Alcohol-induced hypoglycemia results for the toxic effects of ethanol on the liver that is not allowed to release glucose properly
- Maintain your blood glucose levels under control. This will avoid complications

- If you have a mild to moderate hypoglycemic reaction, drink any of the following:

  > 4 oz of any fruit juice or a regular (not diet) soft drink or
  > 8 oz of milk
  > **(4 oz = ½ cup—8 oz = 1 cup)**
  > 1-2 teaspoons of sugar or honey
  > 6 pieces of hard candy.

Check blood glucose in fifteen minutes. If level is below 70, repeat the above suggestions.

- Exercise can lower your blood sugar
- Severe hypoglycemia can lead to unconsciousness. Ask your doctor if you qualify to have glucagon injections. This drug rises the blood glucose quickly and can be administered by a relative at home if you become unconscious
- An identification bracelet is desirable
- If you have frequent hypoglycemic reaction, you may need a change of doses or medications

Normal Blood Glucose Levels (mg/dL)

In people who do not have diabetes

Fasting	70-110
After meals	70-140

In people who have diabetes

Before meals	90-130
One to two hours after the start of a meal	less than 180
Hypoglycemia	70 or below

Tumors

A pancreatic tumor called insulinoma can cause severe hypoglycemia due to excessive insulin production. This tumor is rare and does not usually spread to other areas of the body. There are medical and surgical treatments for this condition.

Death due to hypoglycemia is rare.

For more information, you may contact the following:

American Diabetes Association
National Service Center
1701 North Beauregard Street
Alexandria, VA 22311
phone: 1-800-232-3472 fax: 703-549-6995 e-mail: *customerservice@
    diabetes.org*
Internet: www.diabetes.org

Juvenile Diabetes Research Foundation International
120 Wall Street
19th Floor
New York, NY 10005-4001
phone: 1-800-533-2873 or 212-785-9500 fax: 212-785-0505 e-mail:
    info@jdrf.org
Internet: *www.jdrf.org*

144—HYPOKALEMIA

Hypokalemia means lower than normal serum levels of potassium (K). Potassium is essential for nerve conduction and contractility of the skeletal and cardiac muscle. The normal concentration of K in the serum is in the range of 3.5-5.0 mEq/L (milliequivalents per liter). Hypokalemia exists when serum potassium levels fall below 3.5 mEq/L.

Hypokalemia is most commonly caused by diuretics. These drugs are used in various conditions including hypertension, heart failure, liver and kidney disease. Two of the most commonly used diuretics, thiazide and furosemide, can lead to hypokalemia but other diuretics, such as spironolactone and triamterene, do not produce hypokalemia and in some cases, they have the opposite effect: they retain K in the body and may cause hyperkalemia, high serum K levels.

Diarrhea and vomiting induced by infectious agents cause hypokalemia.

About 2.5 million infants die in the world annually, most of them in the poorer parts of Asia and Africa. In the United States, dehydration is an important cause of K depletion. Since K controls muscle action, the heart muscle may stop beating. Young infants are particularly vulnerable and at risk of death, especially when diarrhea continues for two weeks or longer.

Enemas and laxative abuse, which sometimes are part of an eating disorder (anorexia, bulimia) may lead to life-threatening hypokalemia.

Vomiting may cause hypokalemia but not because the vomited material contains so much K but because the eliminated acid contained in the gastric juice, turns the blood more alkaline and this, in turn, provokes the kidneys to eliminate more potassium.

Alcoholics often have hypokalemia, and it's due to a combination of vomiting, diarrhea, and poor nutrition.

Prolonged fasting and starvation can cause hypokalemia, but it may take a long time to do it. Some people registered 3 mEq/L of serum K after one hundred days of fasting. There are several endocrinological disorders accompanied by hypokalemia. Excessive licorice intake does it too.

SYMPTOMS

Moderate hypokalemia causes leg cramps during exercise, muscle discomfort, weakness, confusion, disorientation. Severe hypokalemia results in extreme weakness of the body and paralysis. Death may occur when the respiratory muscles paralyze or when the heart stops beating. Severe hypokalemia is defined as serum potassium under 2.5 mEq/L.

TREATMENT

Severe hypokalemia is a medical emergency that needs intensive care unit management. It is essential to carefully follow the respiratory and cardiac function. Intravenous K is administered. In moderate cases, oral K supplements can be used (KCl or potassium chloride).

Patients who take diuretics must be checked regularly for signs of K depletion and serum K levels. Not all patients who take diuretics need to be treated with K supplements. When a patient has renal insufficiency, sometimes an excess of K is retained in the blood, and the administration of K can be hazardous.

Patients who have hypokalemia, and at the same take digitalis are at a high risk of digitalis intoxication, and this also requires careful monitoring, at times, in the hospital environment.

Foods with a high content of K include bananas, tomatoes, cantaloupes, figs, raisins, kidney beans, potatoes, and milk.

145—HYPOMAGNESEMIA

This condition means lower than normal blood levels of magnesium (usually a serum level less than 0.7 mmol/L).

What is quite remarkable about this condition is that it is not part of many routine blood tests that include blood count, glucose, calcium, phosphorus, liver function tests, among others, and its deficiency is often undetected. Trouble is that magnesium deficiency can cause death.

Where's magnesium in the human body? This contains 21-28 g of magnesium. Fifty-three percent is located in bone, 19% in non-muscular tissue, and 1% in extracellular fluid such as blood. Some of the magnesium is free and some is bound to proteins, bicarbonate and phosphate.

Magnesium can be found in green vegetables, nuts, wheat, seafood, and meat. It is absorbed in the small bowel although the sigmoid colon and rectum absorb it too to a lesser degree. **This is why high level of magnesium in the blood have been reported following administration of enemas containing magnesium.**

When, for some reason, blood levels of magnesium decrease, the bone reservoir comes to the rescue and releases this important substance.

Lack of magnesium inhibits the release of parathyroid hormone, and this translates into hypocalcemia or low serum calcium.

CAUSES OF HYPOMAGNESEMIA

Ten to twenty percent of all hospitalized patients, and 60-65 % of patients in the intensive care unit have hypomagnesemia. This results from insufficient consumption of magnesium, defective absorption in the gut, or excessive excretion by the kidneys.

Low serum magnesium levels may be due to a long list of disorders. Some of them include the following:

- Acute myocardial infarction
- Acute pancreatitis
- Alcoholism
- Antibiotics
- Excess calcium
- Excess coffee or tea
- Dehydration
- Diabetes
- Diarrhea
- Digitalis
- Diuretics
- Excessive sugar consumption
- Hydrogen fluoride poisoning
- Insufficient vitamins B6, vitamin D, and sun exposure
- Selenium deficiency
- Severe stress

Forty percent of hypomagnesemia also have hypocalcemia (low serum levels of calcium). Sixty percent have hypokalemia (low serum levels of potassium).

TREATMENT

This depends on the degree of deficiency and the clinical effects. Oral replacement is adequate for patients with mild symptoms. Those with severe clinical symptoms require intravenous administration of magnesium sulfate. The disorders that may require intravenous magnesium are the following:

a- Arrhythmias, including malignant tachycardias. Magnesium helps to stabilize arrhythmias that do not respond to other medications
b- Obstetrics: preeclampsia (magnesium reduces vasospasm). Cerebral vasospasm can cause convulsions
c- Acute asthma: magnesium has a bronchodilatory effect

Dying from magnesium deficiency is not only sad. It's tragic since a cardiac arrest can be prevented by suspecting the condition, proving it with a blood test, and replacing it intravenously.

146—HYPOTHERMIA

Two women die the same night and go to the gates of heaven where they'll be evaluated for admission. They start a conversation about their death experiences.

Mary: *Rose, we both died a few hours ago. Did you have pains or discomforts? Was it easy? Was it difficult? Can you tell me?*

Rose: *I sure can! It wasn't really that bad. I remember, I was freezing. I was so cold! Then little by little I became unresponsive and that was it. What about your experience, Mary, how was it?*

Mary: *Oh, sister! Mine was terrible! I had a very rough time! You see, it was midnight, and I had no doubts that my husband had a mistress inside my house, and I went crazy looking for her. I looked all over: inside the closets, under the beds, the bathroom, every place imaginable, but I couldn't find her. My husband pretended to be asleep. I went up and down intensifying the search. Then the stress and the upset reached a critical point, I developed chest pains, an acute heart attack, and here I am!*

Rose: *Mary, I'm so sorry you failed to look inside the refrigerator. Had you done so, there's a good chance that we'd both be still alive!*

Organisms need a certain temperature to live. Normally, humans and other warm-blooded animals maintain body temperature near a constant level through a biological process called homeostasis.

When body temperature drops below what is required to maintain normal metabolism and bodily functions, these become affected. If persistent and unattended, the process may end in death.

Normal body temperature in humans is 37 °C (98.6 °F).

It is estimated that 800 recreational boaters, commercial fisherman, and merchant mariners die each year in the United States as a result of cold water immersion hypothermia. The mortality statistics, however, include many of these deaths as drowning.

Alcohol, diabetes, advanced age, and drug intoxication predispose to more severe degrees of hypothermia. Suicide, psychiatric disorders, and motor vehicle accidents are also contributing factors.

HYPOTHERMIA STAGES

Stage 1—Body temperature drops by 1-2 °C below normal temperature (1-8-3.6 °F). Shivering occurs, hands become numb and are unable to perform complex tasks. Breathing gets shallow and quick. Goose bumps form. The entrance into stage 2 is the person's inability to touch his or her thumb with his or her little finger (the muscles are not working). Panic and shock can place severe strain on the body and a cardiac arrest.

Stage 2—Temperature drops by 2-4 °C (3.6-7.2 °F). Shivering becomes more intense and so does muscular coordination. Movements are slow, stumbling pace; mild confusion; body is pale; lips, ears, fingers, and toes are blue.

Stage 3—Body temperature drops below 32 °C (90 °F). Shivering stops, thinking is sluggish, amnesia appears, and so does the inability to use hands. Below 30 °C (86 °F), walking is difficult to impossible, behavior is incoherent and irrational, arrhythmias develop (fast or slow rates). Most major organs fail to function. Clinical death (no pulse, respirations, blood pressure) occurs although due to decreased cellular activity during stage 3 hypothermia, brain death takes longer.

TREATMENT

Mild hypothermia (some shivering, but the victim can hold a rational conversation) only requires removal of wet clothes and replacement with dry clothes or blankets.

Severely hypothermic patients have a very good chance of survival when treated on time and properly. If a person dies during rewarming, and there is no other trauma or disease, this suggests the individual may have died from inappropriate or ineffective treatment.

The victim should be taken out of the water and provided a warm environment. Remove the clothing only if it can be done with a minimum of movement of the victim's body. **This restriction will minimize additional heat loss. Massage of the extremities should be avoided for the same reason.**

The semiconscious person should be laid face up, with the head slightly lowered unless vomiting occurs. The head-down position allows more blood to flow to the brain.

The first thirty minutes of hypothermia treatment are critical. The primary goal is to stabilize the victim and prevent any further drop in body temperature. It is imperative to start rewarming in the field. In some cases, the victim cannot be mobilized, and rewarming must start on-site.

If available, place the person in a bath of hot water at a temperature of 105-110 °F. **It is very important to keep the arms and legs out of the water to prevent "after drop." After drop occurs when the cold blood from the upper and lower extremities is forced back into the body resulting in further lowering of the body temperature. After-drop can be fatal.**

If a tub is not available, apply hot, wet towels or blankets to the victim's head, neck, chest, groin, and abdomen. **Do not warm the arms or legs.**

If nothing is available, the rescuer can use his or her own body to warm a hypothermic victim.

In short: dry, shelter, and gradually warm the victim. Blankets offer limited help. Close contact with another person and drinking sweet-warm fluids are better options.

Severe cases of hypothermia require immediate treatment in a hospital. Temperature stabilization is through inhalation of warm humidified air or oxygen. The RES-Q-AIR system makes this available for any emergency or rescue operation. This is particularly crucial during the first thirty minutes of hypothermia therapy.

Inhalation rewarming is the only substantiated, noninvasive method of internal rewarming. This method is used in hospitals and other special situations such as caving rescue, mountain rescue, ski resorts, and coast guard for sea rescues.

Active internal rewarming techniques include gastric, thoracic, and peritoneal lavage (circulation of heated solutions in body cavities); diathermy (use of ultrasound and microwave); extracorporeal circulation (circulating and heating of the blood outside the body), heated IV solutions.

Cardiac arrhythmias are more resistant to treatment when the patient is severely hypothermic.

And now, careful about this: There have been impressive cases of recovery after prolonged cardiac arrest in cases of severe hypothermia. This is probably due to the fact that low temperatures prevent cellular damage when blood flow and oxygen supply ceased for an extended period of time. Therefore, a patient should **not be considered dead until he or she is warm and dead.**

Research and real life experiences indicate that people survive cold-water immersion much longer than popularly believed. Many children have been brought up from freezing water after thirty minutes and been successfully resuscitated.

PREVENTION

- Cold water robs the body's heat a lot faster than cold air. Getting out of the cold water as fast as possible by any available means is critical
- Persons boating in the cold-water months should be skilled in rescue and self-rescue techniques. Most accidents involve small boats. Most boats, even filled with water, will support the weight of its occupants. If the boat has capsized and cannot be made right, climb on top of it
- Physical exercise, such as swimming, causes the body to lose heat at a much faster rate than remaining still in the water
- If you find yourself in the water, avoid panic. You'll have to make a decision depending upon the circumstances. If you remain still, you'll delay hypothermia. If you swim, the physical effort will greatly increase heat loss. So it's the kind of catch-22 situation that nobody likes to face
- Always make sure your boat and equipment are in first-class condition. Check the weather forecast before boating. Tell someone where you are going and when you expect to return. Next to the diver's wet suit, wool clothing offers the best protection. Don't forget to wear a personal flotation device (PFD) when boating
- Appropriate clothing helps to prevent hypothermia. What is appropriate? The kind of clothing that does not retain much water from the skin's perspiration. Why? Because water quickly conducts heat away from the body. **Cotton is not good because it retains water. Synthetic and wool fabrics provide more protection because they dry quicker**

- Curiously, the head is the part of the body where most heat is lost (one-third of the body's heat). So it is very important to cover and warm up the head

Children are particularly sensitive to hypothermia. In a couple of hours in water as warm as 16 °C (61 °F), they may die in seawater.

Alcohol and hypothermia make a powerful and nasty cocktail. Alcohol causes generalized vasodilatation, and heat of the circulating blood is lost through the skin more easily. The individual feels warmer when he or she drinks, because the skin vasodilatation brings in more blood. This is a temporary phenomenon that disappears when the heat has dissipated through the skin.

Alcohol-induced hypothermia is one reason for the development of pneumonia. When hypothermia due to other reasons complicates the picture, the prognosis is even more reserved.

Never give alcohol to a hypothermic patient under any circumstances!

THE UNDRESSING PARADOX

Persons who suffer from severe hypothermia become disoriented, agitated, and confused. This behavior leads some of them to remove their clothes, and victims have been found dead before a team came to the rescue. Police have sometimes wrongly assumed that these situations were due to a sexual assault.

Hypothermia may be fatal. However, those who are informed about the best ways of preventing and treating this condition will have better chances of survival if they are ever challenged by this chilling condition.

147—HYPOTHERMIA DUE TO WATER IMMERSION

Cold-Water Survival

Tolerance to low temperatures varies from person to person. The physical condition matters and can make a big difference in cases of cold-water immersion.

The first reaction of a person who suddenly plunged into cold water is one of panic and shock. It may be intense enough to cause an immediate cardiac arrest. Far oftener, the victim gets disoriented, and the extremities become so numb that they cannot be moved. Unless helps arrives quickly, unconsciousness and death will ensue.

Normal body temperature is 97-98.6 °F. A temperature of 96.5 °F will cause shivering. At 94 °F, amnesia; at 86 °F, loss of consciousness; and death at approximately 79 °F.

WHAT TO DO

Those who do boating in the cold-water months should be trained in the skills of rescue and self-rescue. Most accidents involve small boats. Usually, boats filled with water will support the weight of the occupants. If the boat has capsized, try to make it right. If you can't, climb on top of it.

Swimming will significantly increase heat loss from your body and shorten survival time by more than 50%. On the other hand, you might need to make a tough decision and try to swim to get out of the water. The decision is a tough one: either you conserve body heat by not swimming or you don't move and wait for the rescue team.

PRECAUTIONS

- Your boat and equipment should be in perfect condition
- Check the weather forecast before you go boating
- Always tell someone where you are going and when you expect to return
- Wear several layers of light clothing
- Best suit is a diver's wet suit. Wool clothing is the second best
- Wear a personal flotation device (PFD)

FIRST AID

- Get the person out of the water and into a warm environment
- If possible, remove wet clothes with a minimum of movement of the victim's body. This is to avoid heat loss
- Do not massage the extremities
- Lay the semiconscious person face up

- Use warm humidified oxygen by face mask if you know how to do it
- Warm the victim immediately by placing him/her in a bath of hot water at a temperature of 105 °F
- Keep the victim's arms and legs out of the water to prevent "after-drop."

NOTE: After-drop occurs when the cold blood from the limbs is forced back into the body. This results in further lowering of the body temperature and can be fatal.

- If a tub is not available, apply hot, wet towels or blankets to the victim's head, neck, groin, and abdomen
- **Do not warm the arms or legs**
- If nothing is available, a rescuer may use his or her own body heat to warm up the affected person
- Never give alcohol to a hypothermic individual. The vasodilatation alcohol produces, dissipates the body heat and that's exactly the opposite of what you want to do

AND NOW, REMEMBER THE FOLLOWING

Many persons recovered in cold water in "near" drowning condition may look dead and have no detectable breathing, pulse, heartbeat, and are blue (cyanotic) with dilated pupils.

Sometimes, these people are not dead. How may these individuals survive? Because of the "diving reflex" blood gets diverted away from the arms and legs and is shifted to vital organs such as the heart, brain, and lungs. Sometimes, the victim only has six or eight beats per minute. CPR must be provided immediately. Make sure you know what you're doing because if you don't you may worsen the person's already-critical situation. Always be knowledgeable about CPR when you participate in these boating activities. Get properly trained.

Also keep in mind that a number of children have been successfully resuscitated after being immersed in freezing temperatures for twenty minutes.

148—IGNORING WARNING SYMPTOMS

A number of illnesses capable of killing a person instantly or in a very short period of time fire some warning shots and cause symptoms that, when properly recognized, allow for timely corrective action.

Cardiovascular disease is the number one killer in the United States. Sixty-three million people are affected by it. An **acute myocardial infarction** may appear without warning at any time, but it often presents as a chest discomfort that typically feels like a tightness, heaviness, or constriction. Many confused it with "indigestion." Occasionally, the pain is not located in the chest but involves the left shoulder or both shoulders, the left arm, or both arms, the back, jaw, anterior neck, elbows, wrists, upper abdomen or earlobes. Or insidious shortness of breath and newly developed intense fatigue may announce the storm of a coronary event due to a critical obstruction of a coronary artery.

Whenever you experience such symptoms, you've got to consult your doctor *fast*.

Quick recognition of this problem prompts immediate treatment in the hospital setting.

Another symptom that must be paid attention to is **fainting or acute loss of consciousness, also called syncope.** This may be due to relatively benign problem such as low blood pressure induced by medications, emotional upset, or intense fear.

Some other causes that can be potentially fatal:

- Severe **obstructive cardiomyopathy,** a thick heart muscle that blocks the exit of blood from the left ventricle, a cause of sudden death in athletes
- **Cardiac arrhythmias**
- **Critical narrowing of the aortic valve (aortic stenosis)**

These conditions often cause dizziness, fainting, chest pains, or shortness of breath in days, weeks, or months preceding the last catastrophic episode.

* An **acute severe cerebral hemorrhage** (due to the bursting of a cerebral artery) may follow uncontrolled hypertension, and that should be enough to seek urgent effective control of the blood pressure

Any severely hypertensive patient who drinks excessive alcohol is a prime candidate to suffer a cerebral hemorrhage.

* **Acute pulmonary emboli** (clots blocking the pulmonary artery that traveled from the legs) are very dangerous, and just one big clot lodged in the main pulmonary artery may cause an abrupt loss of life. Obese individuals as well as those who never do exercises are prime candidates to suffer this condition and its often dreadful consequences. These clots could be avoided, that is, if the weight is normalized and exercises are practiced regularly.

* An individual who has speech impairment, double vision, loss of vision on one side, confusion, disorientation, or weakness of one arm or leg, any of the above or in various combinations may be announcing an imminent stroke. If the **carotid arteries in the neck are severely or critically narrowed, something needs to be done** rapidly (stent implantation or removal of the atherosclerotic plaque by surgery called carotid endarterectomy) **to avoid a stroke, which could be fatal.**

* Abdominal or back pains may recur for weeks due to an **enlarging abdominal aortic aneurysm (AAA).** The condition is easily diagnosed by an abdominal aortic ultrasound that just takes a few minutes to do.

* Those who have **black tarry stools** must go to an emergency department fast. This is usually due to an acute gastrointestinal bleeding and needs immediate attention, even if after having the black stools you feel well and think that the bleeding stopped. **GI bleedings** are notoriously unreliable and dangerous. I've seen patients having cardiac arrests from massive gastrointestinal bleeding who had had the first black tarry stools at home and hoped that it would never happen again. In the hospital environment, I had to attempt the revival of a victim who turned as pale as a white sheet and had a cardiac arrest while sitting at the toilet, passing blood through the rectum profusely.

* Some **headaches** thought to be due to migraine or stress **may in fact be due to an imminent rupture of a cerebral aneurysm.**

* A **major depression** may not be clearly recognized on time and **suicide** takes relatives and doctors by surprise. Anyone with severe depression needs very urgent attention.

* **Long-standing cardiovascular risk factors may be responsible for a sudden death.** Unfortunately, millions of individuals ignore them or neglect their proper treatment. These will be discussed in a separate section **(section 124).**

Always pay attention to warning symptoms that announce possible stormy outcomes. I constantly see men and women who take great care of their house, car, or motorcycle maintenance, but when it comes to taking care of their health, they fail miserably. And of course, a price is paid for such neglect. Don't fall into that trap!

149—LIGHTNING

I was trimming some plants and bushes in the garden of my house. It was a cloudy day, and it was beginning to rain. I heard the voice of one of my children coming from inside the house that said, "Dad, come on in. There's quite a bit of lightning outside. It's dangerous." I complied with the advice. Seconds after I entered the house, lightning struck the tree I had been trimming, produced a deep cut in the trunk and left it partially burned. Had I stayed in that place for a few more seconds, I would have probably been electrocuted.

Lightning is an electrical discharge that occurs between the ground and clouds or between clouds. The lower part of the clouds are charged negatively and objects on the ground like steeples, trees, and the earth itself become positively charged, creating an imbalance. The result is an electrical current that is produced between these two charges. This can get through a building, a tree, or a person. Most lightning travel from cloud to cloud, but some are discharged and reach the ground.

Lightning is extremely hot. A flash can heat the air around it to temperatures five times hotter than the sun's surface. This heat causes surrounding air to rapidly expand and vibrate, which creates the typical thunder we hear a short time after seeing the lightning flash.

Worldwide, there are 50-100 lightnings per second, and each one contains hundreds of millions of volts. Central Africa and South America have the greatest concentration of lightning. Sixty to one hundred lives are lost every year in the United States due to lightning, and 2,000 people are killed worldwide every year. In USA, another 300 people are injured by this phenomenon, and many of them must deal with lifelong disabilities. In a given year, the chance of being killed by lightning in the United States is about 1 in 700,000, and the chance of being killed by lightning is less than 1 in 6 million. The chance is far less in places where thunderstorms are infrequent (San Francisco) and much greater where thunderstorms are frequent (Central Florida).

In the United States, lightning causes more deaths than do most other natural hazards (e.g., hurricanes and tornadoes). Lightning has struck ten miles away from the rain of a thunderstorm. In the United States, cloud-ground lightning strikes occur thirty million times each year, most often in Florida and along the southeastern coast of the Gulf of Mexico.

Neurological and cardiopulmonary injuries associated with lightning strikes are the most dangerous and life threatening. These may stop the heartbeat completely or produce ventricular fibrillation or affect the respiratory center located in the central nervous system. The heart muscle may suffer an acute, massive dysfunction, and fast accumulation of pericardial fluid may be fatal unless it's quickly treated. Resuscitation of patients who had a lightning-induced cardiac arrest should be initiated without delay.

PRECAUTIONS TO AVOID BEING STRUCK BY LIGHTNING

When a thunderstorm threatens, do the following:

Indoors

- Avoid using the telephone unless you have an emergency. Lightning may strike electric and phone lines
- Don't turn on electrical appliances, TV sets, and computers. Disconnect them
- Remain indoors until the storm has passed
- Keep away from doors, windows, fireplaces, metal pipes, and sinks
- Don't use water during the storm

Outdoors

- Get into a house, a large building, or a hard-top automobile. **No** place outside is safe in a thunderstorm
- Once inside the house, stay off anything that is conductive, such as wiring or plumbing
- Stay away from corded phones. Disconnect computers and TV sets

- Stay away from antennas, fences, electric wires, and train tracks (rails can transmit electricity from a distance)
- Do not take a bath or a shower
- Do not swim in an indoor pool
- Make sure the kids' video game terminals are cordless
- When you hear thunder, go to a safe place and stay there for thirty minutes after the last thunder. Safe places are vehicles with a solid metal top or solid metal sides such as buses, most cars, and trucks
- If you are in your car, stay there
- Avoid elevated places, open areas, and water-related activities: swimming, fishing, boating
- Never stand underneath a tall, isolated tree
- Avoid open spaces
- Stay away from metal items such as antennas, fences, electric wires, and train rails.
- If you are fishing or playing golf, put the rods and the clubs down
- First aid: start CPR immediately and have someone call 911

Be careful and follow these instructions. If you do, you'll likely avoid a disastrous outcome from this powerful force of nature. And don't forget to share with your family and friends what you've learned today.

150—LIVER FAILURE: ACUTE AND FULMINANT

Acute liver failure (ALF) is an uncommon condition in which the liver is affected to the point where survival is not often possible. It is a rapid deterioration that occurs in a previously young and healthy individual. The liver normally manufactures, among many other things, substances that control the blood coagulation. In ALF, this process fails, and severe bleeding tendencies occur. There are also mental alterations (encephalopathy). There is no preexisting liver disease, such as cirrhosis or anything else. This disorder carries a high mortality.

Hepatitis viruses or autoimmune hepatitis and hypersensitivity to many drugs can produce acute and fulminant liver failure (antibiotics such as ampicillin, ciprofloxacin, erythromycin, tetracycline, and others), antiepileptics (phenytoin), anesthetic agents (halothane), salicylates (Reye's syndrome), illicit drugs (ecstasy, cocaine), nonsteroidal anti-inflammatory agents, antidepressants (amytriptyline, nortriptyline), and others, are capable of causing this dreadful complication.

The leading cause of ALF in USA and the United Kingdom, however, is drug-related liver toxicity, and the recognized culprit is a medication that has no significant side effect when taken in the right dose: **acetaminophen.** There has been a dramatic increase in acetaminophen toxicity recently. This drug, ingested in high doses as it happens with suicide attempts, or unintentionally to relieve severe pain, such as 4 g/day far exceeds other causes of acute liver failure in the United States, and usually to susceptible patients and in the context of depression, chronic pain, alcohol or narcotic use.

In the United States, 2,000 cases annually of ALF occur per year, and drugs are responsible in more than 50% of ALF cases. Acetaminophen toxicity accounts for 42%, and 12% of cases are due to other drugs reactions. Nearly 15% of cases remain of indeterminate origin. Other recognized offenders are Hepatitis B virus (HBV), autoimmune hepatitis, Wilson disease, fatty liver of pregnancy, and HELLP (please see chapter 8). Hepatitis E virus (HEV) is associated with high incidence of ALF in women who are pregnant. This is a source of concern when patients live or travel to endemic areas.

THE PATIENT'S FATE depends upon the cause of the disease and the seriousness of the complications. Cerebral edema, renal and respiratory failure, bleeding, and sepsis are difficult to survive, particularly when they occur at the same time. Those who carry a more ominous outlook are younger than ten years and older than forty years. It is important to select those patients who qualify for liver transplantation.

151—MALIGNANT HYPERTENSION DUE TO ANESTHETICS

This is a hypermetabolic response to potent volatile anesthetic gases such as halothane, sevoflurane, desflurane, and the muscle relaxant, succinylcholine.

The incidence of malignant hypertension reactions due to anesthetic is related to a genetic abnormality, and its frequency ranges from 1:5,000 to 1:50,000-100,000 anesthesias. However, the presence of the gene abnormality may be as great as one in 3,000 individuals. Over ninety gene mutations have been identified.

The classic signs of malignant hypertension include marked fever, tachycardia, fast respiratory rates (tachypnea), increased carbon dioxide production, increased oxygen consumption, acidosis, muscle rigidity, and muscular destruction (rhabdomyolisis), all of them related to the hypermetabolic status.

This syndrome tends to be fatal if untreated, so it is crucial to recognize it early. A very helpful sign is to notice an elevation of CO_2 in samples of arterial blood gases.

Dantrolene sodium is a specific antagonist used for anesthesia-induced malignant hypertension, and it should always be available whenever general anesthesia is used. Thanks to a much better understanding of this reactive phenomenon, the mortality rate of this syndrome dropped from over 80% three decades ago to less than 5%.

152—MASSIVE PULMONARY EMBOLISM

At times, one clot that travels to the lung kills faster than two bullets fired into the chest.

The veins of the body are conduits of blood back to the heart. Two large veins, the superior and inferior vena cava, drain the blood into the right side of the heart. From here, the blood is propelled to the lungs for oxygenation.

If the clot remains attached to the vein wall, the patient may have no symptoms or have thigh or calf tenderness and swelling. This is called DVT, deep venous thrombosis. At times, this condition leads to chronic skin changes (ulcerations) and edema (swelling of the leg).

That is, of course, no pleasure to have. But if that clot (thrombus) becomes dislodged from the venous wall and travels to the lungs, the situation may turn into a nightmare. A big clot that blocks a major branch of a pulmonary artery may cause a sudden death. Such cases carry an ominous outlook when they occur in a hospitalized patient treated by the best doctors. If it happens at home, the patient gets brusquely short of breath, and in a few moments he or she is gone.

One clot landing in the lung is a **pulmonary embolus**. Several clots doing the same is termed **pulmonary emboli**. The process is called **pulmonary embolization**.

WHY CLOTS IN THE LOWER EXTREMITIES ARE FORMED?

It is amazing that in 1842, a prominent German pathologist, Dr. Virchow, described three conditions that predispose to clot formation in thighs and legs and that today, his concepts remain scientifically accepted:

- Stasis (sluggish venous circulation)
- Damage to the wall of the vein
- Hypercoagulability (increased tendency to form clots)

SIGNIFICANT RISK FACTORS FOR THROMBOSIS

- Age
- Prolonged physical inactivity
- Cocaine
- Obesity
- Venous insufficiency (over 3-4 % of the population of the United States suffers from chronic venous insufficiency)
- Malignancy
- Recent surgery (particularly lower extremity orthopedic surgery)
- The postpartum period
- Oral contraceptives
- Genetic disorders, including deficiencies of protein C, protein S, protein A, and antithrombin III

A NASTY, LIFE-THREATENING SURPRISE

Pulmonary embolism (PE) is the third most common cardiovascular disease in the United States, after myocardial infarction and stroke. Overall mortality is around 30%. Rates range from 3.5% to 15% and can be as high as 58% when shock is present. Thromboembolic disease is the leading cause of maternal death in the United States. Pregnant women are at increased risk of thrombosis both during pregnancy and postpartum due to a hypercoagulable state (this means the tendency of the blood to form clots).

Early and precise diagnosis of PE is of utmost importance since in 70% of patients who die of the disease, the condition is unsuspected.

Of those who die from PE, 65% of patients do it within one hour of presentation of PE, and 92.9% expire within the first 2.5 hours.

PREVENTION OF DVT AND PE

Prophylactic treatment to prevent DVT and PE is indicated in obese patients and those who are immobile as a result of lower extremity orthopedic surgery, neurosurgery, lower abdominal surgery, trauma or poststroke weakness of the leg. Prophylaxis (prevention) can be mechanical (compression stockings) or pharmacologic (subcutaneous injections of low-molecular-weight heparin).

Anticoagulation with heparin to start with and beginning warfarin while the patient is still in the hospital remain the cornerstone of treatment of deep venous thrombosis (DVT).

DETECTION OF PULMONARY EMBOLI

A few years ago, the ventilation/perfusion (V/P) lung scan was the favorite method to diagnose PE. Although currently other diagnostic methods are considered preferable, still the V/P scan continues to be the safest test and is still the recommended test for patients who are pregnant, nursing, or have moderate-severe renal failure.

There are other diagnostic modalities, and different institutions have placed their trust and confidence in the various scanning machines available.

COMPUTARIZED TOMOGRAPHY OF THE CHEST

Spiral or helical computed tomography angiography. This study is completed in 25-30 seconds. Nearly 90% of patients evaluated for PE are able to hold their breath throughout the study, eliminating motion artifact from breathing.

Multidetector spiral computed tomography. This is an improvement of the above. The use of multiple detectors shortens the time of the study to less than ten seconds and shows greater picture accuracy and visualization.

These tests are not without risks. They are not recommended for patients with preexisting renal disease and pregnancy.

Magnetic Resonance Imaging (MRI)

To date, MRI is not thought to be harmful. It is thought to be safe in pregnant women. In addition there is no organ toxicity due to MRI.

The major concern with MRI for the evaluation of PE is its diminished sensitivity.

There are contraindications for MRI, the most important of which is the presence of an electronic implanted device. Fatal arrhythmias have been attributed to cardiac pacemaker malfunctions during an MRI. So **an MRI should not be done in those who carry a pacemaker.**

Nerve stimulators, continuous medicine pumps, cardiac defibrillators, insulin pumps, cochlear implants, and some prosthetic devices should be considered contraindications as should residual metallic fragments (shrapnel, bullets), which may move during the course of an MRI. Although rare, burns in patients with tattoos have been reported.

There is a blood test called d-dimer. It reflects degradation of blood products, and it shows elevated levels in cases of pulmonary embolism. The test is not specific since d-dimer may show abnormally high levels in other medical conditions as well. However, it is a very sensitive test, which means the following: **if the d-dimer blood levels are normal, the patient does not have pulmonary emboli.**

INTERRUPTION OF THE INFERIOR VENA CAVA (IVC)

When pulmonary emboli (PE) occurs while the patient is being properly treated with anticoagulants or these drugs cannot be given for a number of medical contraindications, a filter is placed in the inferior vena cava (IVC) to stop any incoming clots from the leg or thigh. There are permanent and retrievable filters approved in the United States for the prevention of pulmonary embolism. A typical scenario is a patient who has proven pulmonary emboli and gastrointestinal bleeding at the same time. The bleeding contraindicates the use of anticoagulants for pulmonary emboli. So an IVC filter (inferior vena cava filter) is inserted.

At present, filter insertion is only indicated in patients with proven venous thromboembolism who have an absolute contraindication for anticoagulant therapy, such as high risk for bleeding (intracranial bleed, uncorrected major coagulation disorders, or a spinal cord injury).

When IVC filter is inserted, and unless anticoagulation is contraindicated, anticoagulants must be given as soon as possible.

It must be remembered that filters do not prevent DVT, and in fact, may at times be responsible for recurrent DVT due to blockage of the filter by clots causing its outflow obstruction. And there are a number of additional mechanical failures that filters of this kind occasionally have.

Patients who suffered from pulmonary emboli required oral anticoagulation with warfarin for a period of at least 6-12 months, and at times, warfarin is provided indefinitely.

A fifty-three-year-old cardiovascular surgeon suddenly developed chest pain consistent with typical pulmonary emboli. He had severe varicosities in both lower extremities. This meant sluggish venous circulation and damage to the veins, both of which predispose to venous clot formation.

His hospital course was dramatic. Initially, he had chest pains in multiple sites of both sides of his thorax because he was throwing clots every few seconds. The pains were severe, his pulse was fast, his color purple, his blood pressure low. Anticoagulation did not stop the incoming clots. He was critically ill. An inferior vena cava filter was inserted.

Unfortunately, something went wrong with the filter. It was clogged just a while after its insertion. Hours following this operation, his testicles and lower extremities became severely swollen, edematous, reflecting the filter's failure to let the blood get through to the heart. That translated into total blockage of his inferior vena cava.

This kind of filter was nonremovable. He had a long hospital course and eventually recovered. The blood from the lower part of his body reached the heart through the development of large venous collateral channels.

This condition forced him to give up his cardiovascular surgery practice.

153—MEDICAL ERRORS

Millions of people are regularly saved by health care practitioners and hospitals in the United States. This great country has extraordinary medical centers, researchers, academicians, and practitioners, and they deserve admiration and respect. With that background, one would be inclined to think that errors in medicine occur just occasionally. Regrettably, the statistics show that mistakes of different sorts are frequent and often tragic. Many lives are lost. And the economic impact of medical errors is immense.

The HealthGrades patient safety in American hospital study took a first look at the mortality and economic impact of medical errors and injuries that occurred during Medicare hospital admissions nationwide from 2000 to 2002 (Dr. Chuniliu Zhan and Dr. Marlene R. Miller, *Journal of the American Medical Association* [JAMA], October 2003).

This study supported the Institute of Medicine's (IOM) 1999 report conclusion, which found that medical errors in the United States caused up to 98,000 deaths annually. That was considered a number of epidemic proportions, but the study by HealthGrades found that the IOM data may have underestimated the number of deaths caused by medical errors and that there is little evidence that patient safety has improved in the last five years: an average of 195,000 people in the United States died due to potentially preventable, in-hospital medical errors in each of the years 2000, 2001, and 2002. HealthGrades looked at three years of Medicare data in all fifty states and DC. This Medicare population represented approximately 45% of all hospital admissions (excluding obstetric patient) in the United States from 2000 to 2002.

Dr. Samantha Collier, HealthGrades Vice President of Medical Affairs made this point: "If we could focus our efforts on just four key areas—failure to rescue, bed sores, post-operative sepsis, and post-operative pulmonary embolism—and reduce these incidents by just 20%, we could save 39,000 people from dying every year."

IATROGENESIS

This is damage inflicted to a patient by a health care professional. Now, not every complication of medical treatments is avoidable or due to error or neglect. Radiation and chemotherapy for cancer often result in serious complications (esophageal scarring, baldness, weak cardiac muscle, nausea and vomiting, and profound weakness), but these result from the nature of the treatment and not medical incompetence. Nosocomial infections are the nightmare of the medical profession (*nosocomial* means that the complication occurred in a hospital). Uncleaned and ungloved hands, contaminated urinary catheters, infected needles and intravenous drugs, improper sterilization of surgical instruments all conspire to the great disaster of losing lives by the thousands.

Once in a while, a mentally ill health care professional was responsible for the patient's demise. American physician Richard J. Schmidt tried to kill his girlfriend by contaminating her with AIDS-tainted blood. A German surgeon and professor, Ernst Ferdinand Sauerbruch (1875-1951), became demented and continued to perform operations that made no sense at all and that resulted in his patients' death, but he was so famous and powerful that it took a while to stop him from killing people.

SOME SUGGESTIONS TO AVOID MEDICAL ERRORS

- Have good communication with your doctor
- Don't hesitate to obtain a second opinion if you feel you need it. Second opinions disagree with the first opinion 20% of the time
- If a doctor badly resents your suggestion for a second opinion or consultation, don't trust him/her
- Make sure the recommended surgery or procedure is necessary
- Doctors and nurses must wash their hands before they examine you
- The hospital should have the appropriate number of nurses. Shortages of this kind may translate into poor medical care
- Urinary catheter insertion needs special antiseptic precautions, which are often neglected. A sterile field must be prepared, and the head of the penis must be thoroughly cleansed before the catheter makes contact with the urethral orifice
- If you need insulin coverage, ask the nurse twice if he or she is about to give you the correct doses, and ask how many units of insulin you are going to be injected. An excessive amount may cause dangerous hypoglycemia
- If you've been recommended a procedure or surgery, find out if the benefits outweigh the risks or the risks outweigh the benefits
- If you've been scheduled to have outpatient surgery, make certain that you do not need an extra day or two in the hospital. Due to economics, some patients are discharged too soon after surgery and they are not ready for it
- Choose the right hospital, one that offers the latest and most effective tests and treatments and have the best doctors. Look for hygiene standards
- Choose the right doctor. Dedication, honesty, and competence are all essential. Always try to get board certified specialists

- If your state of health is very delicate or you are an elderly person with health problems and need surgery, do not accept outpatient surgery, which means the discharge from the hospital hours following the operation. You should be kept in the hospital for 1-2 days and be properly monitored

154—MENINGOCOCCEMIA

Many years ago, I worked at a hospital that only dealt with all kinds of serious infections. I saw cases of meningococcemia. It was an impressive, unforgettable sight. The disease is brutal and aggressive!

The germ that causes this illness is the *Neisseria meningititis.* Epidemics were notorious during War World I, World War II, Vietnam and Korean wars. Thousands were involved. Mortality was very high.

Some patients develop spinal meningitis. Others experience sepsis, which consists of an extraordinary number of germs polluting the circulatory system.

The symptoms are high fever, shaking chills, headaches, diffuse muscular pains, nausea, profound weakness, and a rash, which is spread in the trunk, extremities, and eyelids. Then, the so-called petechia appear. These are hemorrhagic lesions in the skin. They are seen all over. There are blood coagulation problems, and other sites of bleeding occur, such as gastrointestinal hemorrhages.

This disorder may announce a catastrophic outcome. Total body collapse is announced by undetectable blood pressure, a profound state of shock from which it is difficult to recover.

TREATMENT
High doses of penicillin

PROPHYLAXIS (PREVENTION)
Rifampin is the drug of choice, 600 mg every twelve hours for two days. And for children, 10 mg/kg every twelve hours for two days. For pregnant women: ceftriaxone 125 mg single intramuscular injection.

The value of prevention in schools or military installation is less certain.

Vaccines are available for bacterial groups A, C, Y, and W-135.

155—MORBID OBESITY

I had followed her medically for four years. She was forty-five and carried 200 lbs of excess weight. Her heart function was normal. Nevertheless, I tried, from the first time I examined her, to encourage her to have gastric bypass surgery and warned her about the risks of having heart failure, a myocardial infarction, or even a sudden death. She was afraid of the possible complications of bariatric surgery. One day, she came to my office complaining of progressive weakness and shortness of breath. Her echocardiogram now showed an extremely weak heart muscle, and the gastric bypass couldn't be done because of it. She died shortly after that.

I discussed this condition in detail in my book ***Morbid Obesity and the Struggle for Survival* by iUniverse, published in 2006.** I wrote a new, an updated version titled ***Morbid Obesity: Will You Allow It to Kill You?*** which is currently in print.

Morbid obesity is defined as a weight excess of 100 lbs or more. This condition has increased incidence of myocardial infarctions, congestive heart failure, strokes, cancer, and sudden death, among many other associated ailments called co-morbidities.

Sudden death may result from malignant arrhythmias, acute myocardial infarction, and pulmonary emboli. The latter condition is due to the release of venous clots in the lower extremities to which obese persons are prone to develop.

Correction of morbid obesity is essential to prevent its serious complications. Special diets rarely succeed, and many patients need to be considered for weight loss surgery (bariatric surgery). Patients who succeed with the surgical treatment of obesity are those who achieve radical behavior modification and are willing to comply **consistently and permanently** with food restrictions, exercise programs, take the necessary vitamins and minerals supplements, and follow-up medical care.

Recently type II diabetes has been noted to regress in about 80% of morbidly obese patients in just a few weeks following bariatric surgery, **before any significant weight loss has occurred.** The reason for this phenomenon is under investigation.

In good hands, bariatric surgery has become a safer proposition due to improved surgical techniques developed in the last several years. For a number of reasons, medical and psychological, this kind of treatment is indicated only for a selected population. Those who qualify for it, though, should be seriously considered.

156—MUSCULAR DISTROPHIES

Boys with progressive, fatal Duchenne's dystrophy rarely have any evidence of myocardial dysfunction before the age of ten years, but by age eighteen all patients have detectable cardiomyopathy. The ventricles become dilated, and SD may occur. Death usually results from respiratory and/or cardiorespiratory failure.

Another muscular dystrophy where SCD due to cardiac arrhythmias is not unusual is myotonic dystrophy. In this condition, two-thirds of the patients have heart disease and also heart failure and arrhythmias.

Several other heritable neuromuscular dystrophies can be associated with cardiomyopathy. The extent of the disease and its outlook varies a great deal. With the currently advanced technology for the treatment of both congestive heart failure and serious arrhythmias, these patients can be successfully treated.

157—NONSTEROIDAL ANTI-INFLAMMATORY DRUGS (NSAIDS)

More than 36 million people take over the counter and prescription NSAIDs for pain relief, mostly headaches and arthritis. Some of them are also included in the formula of bad cold medications. Many consumed them like candy. It is estimated that this results in 103,000 hospitalizations and 16,500 deaths in USA every year.

Many people are still unaware of how serious the complications of taking NSAIDs can be. A list of side effects can be seen on *www.drugs.com*. I'll only mention a few here: chest pains, shortness of breath, slurred speech, balance problems, gastrointestinal bleeding, jaundice, headaches, fever, seizures, stomach pain, chills.

The side effects of these drugs raised so much concern that two new medications of the same category (NSAIDs) Vioxx and Celebrex were most welcome because they reportedly caused less-damaging effect on the stomach lining.

After their release in 1998, these drugs became extremely popular, and they sure relieved many pains, and everybody seemed to be happy. That is, until 2004 when Merck & Co. was forced to remove from the market its drug Vioxx due to the increased risk of heart attacks and strokes associated with this medication.

The National Cancer Society suspended a large-scale study on the possible cancer-preventing effects of Celebrex when subjects were shown to have a higher risk of heart attack. Celebrex remains on the market, but sales have diminished due to concerns about its safety. Pfizer is funding a five-year 100-million-dollar study on Celebrex. European Union countries have declined to participate because of their concern about Celebrex safety.

Millions take NSAIDs for headaches, but in a study published in the *British Medical Journal* showed that patients who took these drugs might be perpetuating their headaches that result from a rebound phenomenon induced by these medications.

Alternatives to NSAIDs are the following:

Bromalain is a natural enzyme obtained from the stem of the pineapple. It blocks the prostaglandins that cause inflammation and pain. It should be taken on an empty stomach.

Curcumin is the yellow pigment of the spice turmeric. It's an anti-inflammatory drug with an action similar to that of NSAID, but it isn't toxic.

Glucosamine and chondroitin: A recent large study by the National Institute of Health (NIH) concluded that glucosamine is as effective as Celebrex in treating moderate to severe knee pain without the side effects.

158—PENETRATING CHEST TRAUMA

Approximately 16,000 deaths per year occur in the United States alone due to chest injuries. Thoracic wounds account for 20-25% of deaths due to trauma. Drug wars, gang rivalries significantly contribute to these numbers.

Wars have been instrumental in providing experience and knowledge about penetrating chest wounds. In fact, the guidelines for treating thoracic trauma were not established until World War II. Other U.S. military interventions contributed to increment surgical knowledge to deal with this kind of trauma. That included Korea, Vietnam, U.S. interventions in Grenada, Panama, the Balkans, Somalia, the Falklands Islands, and the Persian Gulf.

The large metropolitan areas in the United States have a pipeline with the trauma division of major U.S. hospitals due to the abundance of assaults involving firearms, handheld weapons, and impalements resulting from falls or leaps from elevations.

The Impact of a Missile

Any missile entry wound below the nipples (front) and the inferior part of the scapula (back) should be considered to have reached the abdomen.

Missiles from gunshot wounds can penetrate all body regions regardless of the point of entry. Once a projectile enters the thorax, many terrible things may happen. Miracles can happen too: *I once examined a WWII veteran who was in excellent health, and his chest radiograph showed a big bullet inside his lung, very close to the heart but without touching it. He had been wounded during the war, but he was so lucky that the bullet entered his thorax and found refuge in one of his lungs without causing any trouble.*

Mechanism of Injury

Velocity of penetration matters. It can be low, medium, or high velocity. Low velocity includes impalement (e.g., knife wounds). The wounded tissues or organs are just those directly caused by the penetration. Medium injuries include bullet wounds from most types of handguns and air-powered pellet guns, which cause less destruction than wounds caused by high-velocity forces. High-velocity injuries are those produced by bullet wounds of rifles and military weapons.

Penetrations from blast fragments have extremely high velocities and can be very destructive. Mines and grenades can generate fragments with initial velocities of 4,500 ft/s. That is a velocity faster than even most rifle bullets. The penetration itself causes great damage, but there's an additional thermal tissue damage.

What is involved? Every organ inside the thorax may be affected, and the subject is too extensive to be dealt with in this book. Blood accumulation in the thorax (hemothorax); lung contusion or perforation (pneumothorax); diaphragmatic muscle rupture; esophageal and tracheal and bronchial tears; pericardial accumulation of blood (tamponade); cardiac wounds, involving the heart muscle, coronary arteries, and valves; sternal bone and rib fractures. Injury of the aorta, pulmonary artery, fistula or injury created communication between trachea and esophagus, laceration of the superior and inferior vena cavae and their main tributaries, the pulmonary veins, the carotids and subclavian arteries, infections.

There are also frequent associated wounds in the neck and abdomen.

Cardiac injuries. Traumatic cardiac penetration is highly lethal; fatality rates reaches 70-80%. Injuries of the ventricles are more common than atrial injuries. The right ventricle is the most frequently involved.

Diagnostic workup. The following are frequently employed: chest x-ray, ECG, echocardiogram including trans-esophageal echocardiogram, CT scanning, CT angiography. Sometimes conventional angiography, bronchoscopy, and esophagoscopy are needed.

Management. It is complex and best provided at specialized trauma centers. Endotracheal intubation may be needed for those who are not breathing (apnea), in shock, or have respiratory embarrassment. Air that is causing a tension pneumothorax (a collapsed lung) requires the immediate insertion of a large-bore needle for immediate decompression usually followed by a chest tube. Blood volume replacement is indispensable in treating hemorrhagic shock.

The surgical management of thoracic injuries requires great skill, knowledge, and dedication.

159—PERITONITIS

This is an infection of the membrane called peritoneum that lines part of the abdominal cavity and some of the organs it contains. It is generally an acute condition that often results from the rupture of a hollow viscus, characteristically a perforation of the lower esophagus and the stomach (peptic ulcer located in the stomach or duodenum); appendicitis, acute gallbladder disease, inflammatory bowel disease, intestinal infarction (an occlusion of an intestinal artery that deprives a section of the gut from blood supply). This allows the passage of the intestines' germs into the peritoneal cavity, intestinal diverticuli, gastric cancer, intestinal strangulation, colorectal cancer, or a perforated colon during colonoscopy.

And there are additional causes where peritonitis occurs without the perforation of a hollow viscus, such as a surgical wound, abdominal trauma, ambulatory peritoneal dialysis, intraperitoneal chemotherapy, and pancreatitis.

The germs contaminating the peritoneal cavity represent a mixture of bacteria: *Escherichia coli*, *Bacteroides fragilis*, *Staphylococcus aureus*, and fungi, such as *Candida*.

SYMPTOMS

Symptoms of peritonitis are acute abdominal pain, tenderness, and swelling, all of which are aggravated by moving the peritoneum, which is provoked by coughing and flexing the hips. There's a rebound tenderness caused by pressing a hand on the abdomen, which produces pain, and then releasing it, which causes more intense pain. The abdomen appears rigid, and there's also fever and tachycardia, nausea, vomiting, and abdominal distention due to bowel paralysis (this is called paralytic ileus).

TREATMENT

It requires fluid replacement and intravenous antibiotics. Surgery is mandatory and **must be done through an abdominal incision to expose the abdominal cavity and perform a full exploration of the abdomen and lavage of the peritoneum in addition to the correction of the cause that produced the peritonitis.**

This condition cannot be treated with laparoscopic surgery.

OUTLOOK

Even when properly treated and in patients who are healthy otherwise, peritonitis carries a mortality rate of 10%. This rises to about 40% in the elderly or those who suffer a significant underlying illness.

This disease must be treated surgically and *fast*.

160—PNEUMONIA

Pneumonia is a serious infection of the lung. It may affect one area or one of the lung lobes (pneumonia) or produce patches throughout both lungs (bronchopneumonia). The air sacs fill with pus and fluid. This makes oxygen absorption difficult, so the amount of oxygen in the blood diminishes. When this is severe and the lung infection spreads to other parts of the lung and the rest of the body, pneumonia can cause death. In fact, until 1936, pneumonia was the number one cause of death in the United States. The introduction of antibiotics was a blessing and kept the disease under control.

Over the years, I've seen a considerable number of people dying of pneumonia. This disease must be treated with respect. Fatal cases showed a rapid, drastic course, with fever, confusion and disorientation, and respiratory embarrassment. Endotracheal intubation, intensive respiratory care, antibiotics, and supportive measures may fail to change the course of this process. Patients go into shock, and efforts to save them may prove futile. Caught on time and properly treated though, pneumonia can be successfully treated.

All pneumonias do not respond to antibiotics. Viruses do not respond to them. In 2003, the combination of influenza and pneumonia ranked in the United States as the seventh leading cause of death.

Pneumonia has multiple causes. These are the most important:

- Bacteria
- Viruses
- Mycoplasma
- Other infectious agents, such as fungi including pneumocystis
- Chemicals

BACTERIAL PNEUMONIA

The *Streptococcus pneumoniae* is the most common cause of bacterial pneumonia. A vaccine is available. It attacks anyone, from infants to the elderly. Those more prone to develop it are alcoholics, debilitated individuals, post-operative patients, those who suffer from chronic respiratory diseases or acute viral infections. Fever may be as high as 105 °F, mental confusion is common and the nail beds and lips may turn bluish due to low oxygen content in the blood.

VIRAL PNEUMONIA

Half of all pneumonias are thought to be caused by viruses. Most of them are not serious although these may be severe and occasionally fatal. Cough and breathlessness may be severe. In extreme cases, the patient desperately needs air. A complication by a bacteria makes a bad situation worse.

MYCOPLASMA PNEUMONIA

Mycoplasma organisms were discovered during World War II and have some characteristic of bacteria and others that resemble those of the viruses. It is also called primary atypical pneumonia. Its most prominent symptom is cough that appears in violent bursts. It is rarely fatal.

OTHER KINDS OF PNEUMONIA

Pneumocystis carinii pneumonia (PCP) is caused by an organism believed to be a fungus. This pneumonia may be the first sign of illness in many people with AIDS.

Tuberculosis pneumonia is very dangerous, and early treatment is essential.

Rickettsia is an organism between viruses and bacteria and causes Rocky Mountain fever. And there are other bacteria, viruses, and fungi capable of causing pneumonia.

TREATMENT

It must be provided quickly. The specific antibiotic to be used depends upon the existing type of pneumonia. Antibiotic therapy must last as long as it is considered necessary but **should not be discontinued too soon. Relapses of pneumonia can be far more serious than the first attack.**

Some patients can be treated at home. Others need careful monitoring in the hospital. Appropriate diet and oxygen to increase its level in the blood may be necessary. Adequate rest and nutrition are very important.

PREVENTION

Pneumonia is a frequent complication of influenza (flu). So get the flu vaccine shot every fall.

A vaccine is also available to help fight pneumococcal pneumonia. Ask your doctor if you or a relative qualifies for this vaccination. It is usually given only to people at high risk of getting the disease and its dreadful complications. These include patients with chronic lung or heart disease, diabetes, sickle cell anemia, kidney disease, or those who are recovering from a serious illness, are sixty-five years of age or older and who are living in nursing homes or other chronic care facilities.

The vaccine is not recommended for pregnant women or children under age two.

If you feel you have symptoms of pneumonia (fever, cough, marked weakness, shortness of breath), call your doctor right away. **Do not ever delay the treatment of pneumonia.**

161—POISONING

Poisons are substances that cause injury, illnesses, or death. A poison is different than a venom. Poisons are toxins absorbed through the skin or the gut. They can be biological, such as bacterial proteins that cause botulism and tetanus. Venoms are biological toxins that are injected subcutaneously, by sting or bite.

Millions of people are accidentally poisoned in their own homes. In reality, 90% of poisonings happen in the home. Most of them happen to children between the ages of six months and five years.

The use of poisons. Rapid death by the administration of a poison has been used as a method of assassination, suicide, and execution. The

Greek philosopher Socrates carried a death sentence by swallowing a poison. Carbon monoxide inhalation is often used to commit suicide; legal executions involve the breathing of hydrogen cyanide (gas chamber) or a lethal combination of intravenous substances.

Acute poisoning is exposure to a poison one time or during a short period of time. Contact or absorption of poisons used in warfare can cause rapid death. They can quickly reach the nervous system and are able to paralyze a person in seconds.

Most pesticides are poisons that target organisms. Unfortunately, children are often victims of their accidental ingestion.

IMPORTANT POINTS ABOUT POISONING AND CHILDREN

- Children younger than five years of age and adolescents are prone to poisoning
- Ninety percent of poisonings occur at home, usually the kitchen and the bathroom
- Poisons must be labeled, locked, and out of the reach for children
- Keep all plants out of the reach of small children
- Know the names of your plants and which ones are poisonous
- Grandparents should be careful. Sometimes, they take medications that can be reached and swallow by children
- Keep medications in locked cabinets
- Return medications to safe storage after use
- Never tell children that medicine is candy
- Never take medications in front of children. They like to imitate adults
- Know where the children are at all times and what they are doing. If they are very quiet, check on them
- Parents and those who share the household should always be prepared to call a poison center on emergency basis for quick advice. **In the United States, the number is 1-800-222-1222. Poisons centers in the USA provide immediate, free, and expert advice over the telephone twenty-fours hours a day, seven days a week**

POISONOUS PRODUCTS

Kitchen. Ammonia, carpet and upholstery cleaners, cleaning fluid, cleansers and scouring powders, drain cleaner, furniture polish, metal cleaners, powder and liquid detergents, rust remover, vitamins

Bedroom. Cologne/perfume, cosmetics, medications

Garage, basement, workshop. Antifreeze, arts and crafts supplies, adhesives/glues, fertilizer, gasoline and oil, kerosene, lighter fluid. Lime, cement, mortar, paint, remover and thinner, pesticides/garden sprays, turpentine, windshield cleaner

Bathroom. Aftershave, bath oil, deodorant, hair dyes, hair remover, nail polish and remover, permanent wave solution, room deodorizer, rubbing alcohol, shampoo, shaving lotion, toilet bowl cleaner

General. Alcoholic beverages, batteries, flaking paint

Closets, attic, storage places. Mothballs and sprays; rat, mouse, and ant poisons

Purse. Cigarettes, cigarette lighters, medicines, perfume

Laundry. Bleach, bluing, dyes, disinfectants, powder and liquid detergents, stain removers. Most of these accidents can be prevented. Watch your child and your pet carefully at all times.

There are products that are considered hazardous waste, and you need information on how to proceed with their disposal. Your county health department should be able to advise you on that. Other products can be put in the garbage. Some can be flushed down the toilet or poured down the drain, diluted with lots of water. Read the instructions on their disposal or contact the county health department for assistance.

FIRST AID

- If the poison is an inhalant, remove the victim to a fresh air area
- If the poison made contact with the skin, remove the clothing and wash the skin thoroughly unless a dry power is the cause of the poisoning
- If the eye is affected, flush it abundantly for at least fifteen minutes
- If the poison is ingested, do not induce vomiting and provide small amount of fluids for corrosive agents (e.g., household cleaners)
- Following these measures, call the poison center immediately. You'll be told what to do next

A poison victim must go to a hospital ER. It is essential to deal with cardiopulmonary problems, pain, seizures, or shock.

162—PSYCHIATRIC POLYPHARMACY

Protection & Advocacy Inc. (PAI) is an independent, private, nonprofit agency that protects and advocates for the rights of persons with disabilities, including psychiatric disabilities. Under federal and state law, PAI has the authority to investigate incidents of abuse and neglect of persons with disabilities.

This organization has conducted investigations of death related to the combined use of multiple psychiatric medications. Several cases were reviewed by experts who were critical of the polypharmacy regimen prescribed and the patients' management in the face of their clinical deterioration. Days lapsed between physician visits, medication lists were not reviewed, drug levels were not ordered, medical workups were not conducted.

The primary reason a person receives more than one medication is because administration of a single medication (monotherapy) is ineffective.

Experts and researchers agree that the concurrent use of multiple psychiatric drugs increases the likelihood of unanticipated adverse effects, including death. When multiple medications are used in high doses, cumulative effects may occur that can be dangerous for some patients.

If it is medically concluded that polypharmacy is warranted in an individual case, careful monitoring for possible toxic adverse drug interactions is essential.

High doses of psychotropic medication may cause confusion and delirium. These very same symptoms can be seen in a psychotic patient. At times, it may be difficult to identify the culprit: is the psychosis responsible for this response, or is it the medication or medications prescribed to control the psychotic state and reactions?

One of the cases reported by Protection & Advocacy Inc. was that of a patient who was on a bunch of antipsychotic medications and died. An autopsy was performed, and the county coroner listed the cause of death as "probably adverse reaction associated with multiple drug therapy." The patient was oversedated and obese, and the multiple drugs contributed to respiratory failure. He was a young man who had been admitted two weeks prior to his death.

The likelihood of death is directly proportionate to the number of medications a person with a psychiatry disorder is taking. One study found an increased risk of mortality in persons with schizophrenia with the use of more than one antipsychotic medication concurrently.

Researchers attribute the increased mortality to the cardiovascular effects of many psychiatric medications and the interaction between these medications and other medical conditions, such as cardiac and respiratory disorders. The author of the study concluded: "The greater the maximum number of anti-psychotics given concurrently, the shorter was patient survival.

163—PULMONARY HYPERTENSION

This is the name given to high blood pressure inside the arteries that supply blood to the lungs, the multiple branches of the pulmonary artery. The increased pressure in the pulmonary arterial vessels results from blockages of these vessels due to clots that traveled from the lower extremities (pulmonary emboli).

Thickening of the wall of the arterial branches or their constriction sometimes occur **without known cause. This is called primary pulmonary hypertension,** a serious progressive disease that may lead to a cardiac arrest. There are new drugs to treat pulmonary hypertension that provide some relief. Some congenital cardiac anomalies and diseased cardiac valves may also be associated with pulmonary hypertension. The treatment and outlook varies from case to case.

164—RABIES

I had just graduated as MD and worked at Buenos Aires Medical School, Muniz Hospital. I treated all kinds of infectious diseases in that wonderful and inspiring teaching hospital. During those days, all cases of rabies ended in death. The disease equated to a death sentence. It carried 100% mortality. Today, the disease is still very serious, but the prognosis somewhat improved, that is, if you provide excellent supportive treatment.

CLINICAL MANIFESTATIONS

Rabies begins with flulike symptoms: muscular aches, sore throat, nausea/vomiting, fatigue, headaches. Then, the victim becomes excited and agitated, confused; he/she is combative, has bizarre behavior and hallucinations. Typically, this mental state alternates with lucid periods although these get shorter and shorter. Hydrophobia (increased sensitivity to water) is extreme. I once saw a patient who became extremely agitated and violent when he heard a few drops of water coming out of a faucet. There's also increased sensitivity to light, increased salivation, lacrimation, and perspiration. Cranial nerves cause facial paralysis, double vision, and inability to swallow. Then, coma comes into the picture, and the patient survives an average of four days. With intensive supportive management, some victims survive.

I remember to have seen patients proven to have rabies who presented in coma. The picture was indistinguishable from any other kind of encephalitis. What lead us to diagnose rabies was the history of an animal bite.

PREVENTION

More than 1 million Americans are bitten by animals every year. When should one provide rabies prophylaxis?

The following must be considered:

- Did the individual come into physical contact with saliva likely to contain the rabies virus?
- What animal did the biting? In the United States a bite by a bat that then escapes should receive post-exposure prophylaxis
- What are the circumstances surrounding the exposure?

Any animal suspected of having rabies or any animal that bites unprovoked or exhibits abnormal behavior or is suspected of being rabid should be captured, if possible.

A wild unvaccinated animal, involved in an unprovoked bite, exhibiting abnormal behavior, or is suspected of being rabid should be humanely killed, and the head should be sent to a special laboratory for rabies examination (the FA test, the fluorescent antibody test). If the examination of the brain by this method is negative, it can be assumed that the animal's saliva does not contain the rabies virus, and the exposed person does not need to be treated.

When a wild animal has escaped (foxes, raccoons, bats, skunks, coyotes, etc.) in an area that is suspected or known to have rabies, the victim should receive both passive and active rabies immunization.

If a healthy dog or cat bites a person, the animal should be captured and confined for ten days. If abnormal behavior or any illness develops in the animal during the observation period, it should be killed for FA analysis. It is generally accepted that if the animal has survived without any problems for ten days, it has not transmitted rabies at the time of the bite.

THE DECISION TO PROCEED WITH PROPHYLAXIS

WHAT TO DO

- Treatment of the wound. Scrub the wound with generous amount of soap and water. That will flush the rabies virus
- Clean the wound with 1-4% benzalkonium chloride or 1% cetrimonium bromide. These substances inactivate the rabies virus
- Administer antibiotics and tetanus toxoid
- **Passive immunization with human rabies immune globulin (HRIG)**
- **Active immunization with antirabies vaccine**

PREEXPOSURE PROPHYLAXIS

Individuals with a high risk of contracting the rabies virus: veterinarians, laboratory workers, animals handlers, cave explorers should receive prophylactically the rabies vaccine.

One day, in the midst of a rabies epidemic, a twenty-year-old boy, who had been bitten by a dog, was brought to the hospital with extreme agitation, threatening to bite anyone on sight. Foam came out of his mouth. We diagnosed rabies. So we gave him sedatives, restrained him, and waited for him to die fast, the way all cases of rabies did in the 1960s. After four days, he was still alive. At the end of one-week hospitalization, he continued to be alive. That meant to us that he did not have rabies. It turned out to be a paranoid schizophrenic who had faked rabies. He had learned about the rabies epidemic in town and decided to play the victim's role. So he fooled some people for sometime, but he couldn't fool all the people all the time.

165—RADIATION POISONING

Radiation is medically used to kill cancer cells. These are among the fastest-dividing cells in the body and may be destroyed by a radiation dose that neighboring normal cells are likely to survive. Sometimes, the same ability of radiation to disturb the growth of cancer cells acts in a negative way and causes a malignancy.

Radiation sickness is generally associated with acute exposure. Symptoms are more serious with high doses of radiation. A short exposure can result in acute radiation syndrome. Chronic radiation syndrome requires a prolonged high level of exposure.

MEASURING RADIATION DOSAGE

Doses of radiation are defined in terms of the energy actually deposited in the affected tissue. The symptoms of radiation sickness become more serious (and the chances of survival decrease) as the dosage of radiation increases. Doses are measured in units called sieverts (Sv).

0.05-0.20 Sv: dose exposure causes no symptoms
6-10 Sv: acute radiation poisoning causes near 100% fatality after fourteen days. Bone marrow is destroyed, and the affected person needs bone marrow transplantation.
10-50 Sv: Acute radiation poisoning causes 100% fatality after seven days. Symptoms start in 5-30 minutes, and a few days later, there's massive diarrhea, dehydration, delirium, shock. Death is currently inevitable.

NUCLEAR ACCIDENTS

You would think that nuclear technology and the way governments take care of nuclear materials, reactors, and bombs, accidents in handling them are rare. But that's not the case. In fact, there have been **hundreds of them,** and the gravity of the consequences varied. Some of them were disastrous (see Chernobyl below). Others could have been disastrous.

To give you an overall idea of the kind of incidents involving nuclear material, I'll list just a few:

January 3, 1961: Explosion of a reactor Idaho Falls (USA), killing three people

January 13, 1964: A B-52 plane crashes with nuclear bombs on board in Maryland (USA).

February 6, 1974: Explosion and radiation leak at Leningrad nuclear power plant, three people killed (Russia).

January 14, 1969: USS *Enterprise*, nuclear aircraft carrier, suffers fires and explosions, killing 28 crew members

February 1, 1982: Release of 100 cubic meters of radioactive water from Salem nuclear power plant (USA)

February 9, 1991: Rupture of steam generator pipe causes release of radioactivity at Mihama nuclear power plant (Japan)

February 23, 1981: Accidental explosion of a Pershing II missile (Germany)

February 24, 1972: Accident on board Soviet nuclear-powered submarine causes vessel to lose all power

March 10, 1956: A B-47 plane disappears with nuclear weapon on board in the Atlantic Ocean

March 21, 1984: Soviet nuclear submarine collides with U.S. aircraft carrier *Kitty Hawk*

March 10, 1963: U.S.-nuclear submarine sinks with 123 crew members in the Atlantic.

March 21, 1964: U.S. satellite disperses 1.2 kg of plutonium into the atmosphere

May 22, 1957: Human error causes B-36 plane to release a nuclear bomb in New Mexico

June 1978: Release of two tons of radioactive steam from Brunsbuettel nuclear power plant (Germany).

And there were many other nuclear plant reactor dysfunctions, cooling systems, spilling of nuclear material into the sea, sunken atomic submarines, failures of emergency systems, unwanted ignitions, crew members killed by radiation release, explosion and steam leakage killing workers, and meltdown of reactors.

The worst civilian nuclear accident occurred on April 26, 1986, when a reactor overheated and exploded at Chernobyl nuclear power plant. It immediately killed fifteen people. The most obvious long-term health impact was thyroid cancer that affected approximately 4,000 people, and thousands more are expected to die of cancer. The disaster released at least 100 times more radiation than the atom bombs dropped on Hiroshima and Nagasaki. Much of the fallout was deposited in Ukraine and Russia. Scandinavia and the UK were badly affected by the spread of the radioactive material.

DURING A NUCLEAR WAR

In a nuclear warfare, a person can be irradiated by three processes and these cause burns:

- Thermal burns from **infrared heat radiation**
- **Beta burns** resulting from the fall out particles, which are large and have little penetration into the human body
- **Gamma burns** from highly penetration radiation particles. Patients develop burns to their skin between the time of irradiation and death

DEATHS DUE TO IMPROPER HANDLING OF NUCLEAR MATERIAL

Mishandling of radioactive and nuclear materials lead to radiation release and radiation poisoning. The majority of accidents involve smaller industrial radioactive sources, such as those used in radiography. However, most deadly accidents have occurred due to the mishandling of larger sources used for medical purposes.

We described above the burns produced by radiation. Alpha radiation normally does not penetrate the skin, but the exposure can be much more dangerous after ingestion or inhalation.

THE MYSTERIOUS DEATH OF ALEXANDER LITVINENKO

I can't help it! This sad and tragic story always reminds me of a James Bond movie: the spies' intrigues, the dangers, the double-crossers, and the eternal struggle to survive another day.

If you want to know about rapid death due to radiation poisoning, the case of Alexander Litvinenko will serve you well. Deliberate poisoning was very strongly suspected here. On November 2006 he was poisoned with a radioactive substance, polonium 210.

Litvinenko was a former spy of the Russian security service (FSB). His last job with the agency was heading up the anticorruption unit. He did a good job. In fact, he did such a good job discovering the extent of corruption, that in the process, he created lots of enemies. He was forty-three.

Who ordered the killing? So far, nobody knows for sure.

PREVENTION OF RADIOACTIVE INJURIES

Radiation sickness is prevented by minimizing the dose of radiation exposure, shortening the time of exposure, and getting as far as possible from the radiation site. **Shielding** may be useful if done properly, and it is done by placing a layer of a material that will absorb the radiation between the source and the human. The dose of radiation can be reduced. However, shielding can be tricky because some materials can increase the radiation exposure instead of decreasing it. Details about shielding against radiation are very technical and go beyond the scope of this book.

PROTECTION DURING A NUCLEAR WAR

Death from an atomic bomb first comes from the blast effects. Considerably fewer fatalities seem likely to result from the second-ranking danger, fallout radiation. The atomic bomb dropped in Hiroshima produced a firestorm that burned most buildings within an area of about 4.4 square miles. Many of these fires resulted from the heat radiation from the fireball.

During an atomic explosion, people inside the shelters do not suffer oxygen deprivation but may be killed by carbon monoxide intoxication resulting from the fire's toxic smoke.

Heat radiation ignites fires, and this in turn will set fire to ignitable materials—dry newspapers, upholstery, dry leaves. In war times, sometimes people had to make a difficult choice: to stay inside a shelter where surrounding fires produced carbon monoxide (CO) and penetrated the premises or run outside and suffer a worse death from falling bombs. In those cases, it is useful to have a carbon monoxide detector. If it registers deadly concentration of CO and there's no time to reach another shelter, the occupants should close all openings as tightly as possible, hoping the deadly concentrations of CO will not reach them.

Having said that, I'll move in to the next cause of sudden or rapid death, hoping that human beings will find ways of avoiding wars and settle their disputes by playing video games.

166—RESPIRATORY FAILURE

The air exchange that gives us life occurs in tiny air sacs in the lungs called alveoli. Oxygen is transported from the alveoli to the blood, and this nourishes body tissues and organs. It is the fuel that feeds the body's metabolic activities. A waste product is the production of CO_2 (carbon dioxide) that moves from the blood into the alveoli. So as much as oxygen is absorbed in the lungs, carbon dioxide is eliminated through the lungs.

When the gas exchange is faulty, there is not enough oxygen in the blood (hypoxemia). In addition, there's also accumulation of CO_2 (hypercapnia). This makes the blood acidic. An acid excess (acidosis) injures the body cells and damages the heart and the central nervous system.

CAUSES OF RESPIRATORY FAILURE

There are pulmonary and extrapulmonary causes of respiratory failure (RF). When RF is severe, it can be fatal unless it is properly treated.

These are some examples:

- Asthma or COPD (chronic obstructive pulmonary disease) or emphysema
- Overdose of sleeping pills and/or other legal or illicit drugs
- A premature baby who weighs less than 3 lbs
- A baby with bronchopulmonary dysplasia
- Hyaline membrane disease or respiratory distress syndrome (RDS): this is the commonest respiratory illness affecting premature babies (not having enough surfactant, a substance that makes it possible for air to pass into the alveoli by lowering surface tension and preventing their collapse)
- AIDS pneumonia
- Other pneumonias
- Cystic fibrosis
- Multiple injuries
- Extensive burns
- Severe bleeding

- Sepsis (severe blood infection)
- Morbid obesity
- Exposure to toxic gases, steam, heat during a fire

DIAGNOSIS OF RESPIRATORY FAILURE

It is impossible to estimate the degree or extent of hypoxemia and CO_2 retention. This is accurately done by determining O_2 and CO_2 content in the arterial blood. RF generally means that the O_2 is less than 60 mmHg and CO_2 greater than 45 mmHg.

TREATMENT OF RESPIRATORY FAILURE

It must be provided in an intensive care unit. **No other place is adequate.** Oxygen is administered by mask, nasal prongs, or endotracheal intubation. This latter modality involves the insertion of a tube into the trachea. It allows for removal of secretions by a suctioning machine and the use of mechanical ventilator that will deliver the precise amount and concentration of oxygen.

167—SCORPION STING

In many underdeveloped tropical countries, scorpion stings represent a major public health problem. For every person who dies of snake venom, ten are killed by dangerous scorpions. In the United States, four deaths from scorpion stings were recorded in an eleven-year period. In other countries, such as Mexico, the numbers of victims is much higher.

There are 1,500 scorpion species. Fifty are dangerous to humans. They exist in the Mediterranean countries, Western and Southern Africa, Asia, Central and South America, Caribbean countries, Mexico, and the United States. Scorpions usually hide in cracks and measure from 1 to 20 cm in length. They have their natural habitats (desert and jungle areas), temperate and tropical climate, but sometimes they are forced to change it. This happens when they get into the travelers' luggage, boxes, shoes, and underwear. When you visit a country known to harbor scorpions, always make sure that when you put on an underwear, a scorpion is not taking a nap inside it.

Contrary to popular belief, scorpions are not aggressive. They like to be awake at night and don't hunt for their prey. Their strategy is to wait for an opportunity to strike. Accidental human contact occurs when scorpions are touched while in their hiding places. Most stings involved hands and feet. Their stinger injects the venom, which is usually 0.1-0.6 mg. Sometimes, they sting the victim several times. The toxicity of the venoms depends upon the specie. At times it's mild. Others kill within an hour.

Most deaths occur during the first twenty-four hours after the sting and are secondary to respiratory or cardiovascular failure or a super-acute anaphylactic allergic reaction (please see anaphylaxis). Children are at greater risk because of their lower body weight.

A person who has been stung by a scorpion usually has four signs: mydriasis (large pupils), nystagmus (quick movements of the eye globe), excessive saliva production, unusually marked restlessness, and difficulties to swallow (dysphagia).

FIRST AID

- Use an ice bag to reduce pain and slow down the absorption of the venom (cold produces vasoconstriction)
- Apply a compressive wrap but not too tight
- Move patient as soon as possible to a medical facility. Here, treatment is provided with tetanus prophylaxis, antibiotics if there's an infection, intravenous to treat dehydration and vomiting. Oxygen, intubation, and a respirator are sometimes necessary. The best drug therapy is a combination of a beta-blocker and a sympato alpha blocker. Antivenin is the treatment of choice after supportive care has been implemented

For consultation, call the Arizona Poison Control 602-253-3334. Antivenom lists, location, types, and amounts are available by the joint publication by the American Association of Poison Control Center and the American Zoo and Aquarium Association.

168—SCUBA DIVING

Diving isn't a new discovery. It has been used for fun and other endeavors.

In ancient times, divers sabotaged enemy vessels by boring holes in the ships' hulls. The Greeks constructed complicated underwater defensive shields to protect themselves against attackers. History has recorded that in 1000 BC, a fisherman dove 100 feet, using a rock to accelerate the process of submersion. To do what? To collect sponges!

In WW II, the Italian and the American divers had underwater missions, and their appearance led to their description as "frogmen."

The recreational use of scuba diving and the diving industry followed the publication of a book by Cousteau in the 1950s. And adventurers, looking for gold from ships that sunk centuries ago, explorers and scientists doing marine research use the new technology of scuba diving to achieve their objectives.

WHAT YOU MUST KNOW PRIOR TO SCUBA DIVING

Scuba diving can be dangerous. It may be a great sport, but like any other sport, is not for everybody. You've got to learn what scuba diving is all about and then decide if you really want to become involved with it. In other words, it is a risky sport, and you need to make sure you understand that.

Years ago, a well-known Miami radiologist went for a scuba diving weekend and did not come back alive. I also had a Vietnam veteran who had paralysis of both legs and permanent disability because he developed "bends" when the gas bubbles released during his ascent damaged his spinal cord. The doctor was in his early forties. The veteran was in his early thirties.

THE TOP THREE DANGERS OF SCUBA DIVING

• BAROTRAUMA

It is a pressure-related injury to organs that contain air spaces, e.g., lungs, ears. If you climb up a mountain, it's more difficult to breathe at the top than when you are at the bottom. Why? Because there's less air pressure. In space, there's no pressure; you can't breathe. That's why the astronauts have special suits.

Now when you go underwater, the reverse happens. Water is denser than air and exerts more pressure. The deeper you go, the more pressure you get. So, when you reached a certain depth, your lungs are compressed by the pressure exerted by the water. As you proceed to move up toward the surface, that pressure decreases and the lungs expand. The rapid expansion may cause rupture of the lung tissue and that creates a big problem.

This problem occurs when the diver goes up too fast and doesn't let the air out on his/her way to the surface. **Never hold your breath when scuba diving.** The lungs overexpand while underwater and bursts.

Take a balloon filled with air at 35 ft. When you bring it to the surface, it will explode.

The ear is the most common barotrauma of scuba diving. The resulting earache is known as the "squeeze," and it can be severe. Divers do "clearing" or popping of the ears, and they try to equalize the pressure inside their ears by pinching their nostrils with pressing thumbs underneath the mask and gently blowing through the nose. By doing this, the air will go up to the middle ear and equalize the pressure of the water outside.

- **DECOMPRESSION SICKNESS**

When you have an unopened bottle of Seltzer water, the content looks like water. If you shake it, you'll see bubbles going to the surface. If you open the bottle, the bubbles will continue gargling until all the gas is released.

Apply this to scuba diving: imagine you are the bottle of Seltzer water. If you go underwater and then come up to the surface too quickly, bubbles will form in your blood, and these will go to many different parts of your body. If you come slowly, the bubbles will not form. These bubbles are pressurized in deep water, and as you ascend toward the surface, the nitrogen gas bubbles are released and may cause serious damage. Depending upon their number, size, and location, they are capable of causing a stroke, a heart attack, or paraplegia if the spinal cord got involved. These complications from released gas bubbles is called the "bends."

RECOMMENDATIONS

These were selected from various expert sources including the American Academy of Family Physicians and the DAN (Divers Alert Network).

- To do scuba diving, you have to have a great sense of responsibility
- You should never do scuba diving unless you are fully trained to do it. Get trained through certified classes of scuba diving. In the United States, the two major certification bodies are National Association

of Underwater Instructors (NAUI) and Professional Association of Dive Instructors (PADI). Some courses last 3-4 days, but performance standards and not hours of instruction determine a shorter or longer instruction course

- Keep yourself updated about the marine life around the region you'll use and the risk involved there
- Make sure the equipment is of high quality and in good condition
- Never dive alone
- Dive with a companion who has more experience than you do
- Never ascend too quickly to the water's surface
- Never drink alcohol before a dive
- Consult a doctor if you have any medical conditions, e.g., hypertension, heart disease, seizures, diabetes, hypoglycemia, panic disorder, mental disorder, lung disorders, history of fainting spells, and other conditions. Always make sure your doctor gives you the medical authorization to dive
- Consult your physician about your medications and your safety during diving.
- If you don't feel well or have any kind of pain after your dive, get to the nearest emergency room
- Gently equalize your ears as you descend
- Avoid scuba diving if you are suffering from colds, allergies, infections, or if you took a drug that made you somnolent
- To do scuba diving, you need a good presence of mind and the ability to handle situations without panicking
- Mask and flippers must fit properly
- Educate yourself on your many options to get your diving equipment before you begin shopping
- Ask an expert for advice for quality gear
- Know the weather forecast and the current beneath and the water conditions of on the date of the dive
- Sharks and other large fish account for almost none of the one hundred scuba deaths that occur each year, according to the Diver's Alert Network (DAN). Most shark attacks occur when the victims are standing or swimming in water close to the shore. Nevertheless, it is a good idea to acquire knowledge on how to deal with an unprovoked shark attack. I once went through that experience, and believe me, it wasn't funny at all! (I related that incident in "Shark Attack" (see section 173)

169—SELENIUM DEFICIENCY

Inadequate dietary consumption of selenium is capable of causing a cardiomyopathy that is known as Keshan disease. This was discovered in regions of China whose soil is low in selenium content.

Whether the cardiomyopathy results from the actual selenium deficiency or the selenium deficit increases susceptibility to certain viruses that attack the heart is not clear. Experiments in mice injected with Coxsackievirus B3 show no cardiac effects in those animals with good reserves of selenium. Selenium-deficient mice injected with the virus developed severe myocarditis.

Heart disease (cardiomyopathy) of selenium deficiency can be acute or chronic. The acute form shows severe heart failure, shock, and deadly arrhythmias. Supplemental administration of selenium has a dramatic positive result.

Low selenium levels have been also reported in humans who have been receiving total parenteral nutrition.

170—SEPSIS

Sepsis means a profuse number of bacteria circulating in the bloodstream. Sepsis cases in the United States are estimated to be between 300,000 and 500,000 per year. More than 100,000 are fatal. Two-thirds of the cases occur in hospitalized patients.

A freak accident may ignite the fire of an incredibly rapid loss of life.

When I was a medical student I attended the morgue and was assigned to a team that performed autopsies.

Another student got stuck with a needle he was using to suture some tissue. The cadaver he was working on had died of sepsis. The medical student died in thirty-six hours of fulminant septicemia. He was twenty years of age.

FACTORS THAT PREDISPOSE TO SEPSIS

- Diabetes
- Lymphoma
- Liver cirrhosis

- Burns
- Invasive procedures
- Vascular catheters
- Immunosuppressants
- AIDS
- Decubitus ulcers
- Patients receiving steroids
- Urinary catheters
- Mechanical ventilators
- Intravenous drug injection
- Severe neutropenia (low blood count of white cells called neutrophils)

RECOGNITION OF SEPSIS

Abrupt onset of fever, chills, fast pulse and respiration, altered mental status, and low blood pressure are characteristic. However, in some cases the temperature may be normal or even lower than normal. Absence of fever is more common in infants, in elderly patients, those who have renal failure or alcoholism.

COMPLICATIONS

These are multiple, but the most lethal are septic shock, cardiac and respiratory failure, renal failure, coagulation abnormalities and the disseminated intravascular coagulation syndrome (please see DIC section 129).

DEFINITE DIAGNOSIS

This is established by positive blood cultures that indicate the type of bacteria responsible for the sepsis and what antibiotics these bacteria are sensitive to.

TREATMENT

This includes appropriate intravenous antibiotics for several weeks and removal of the source of the infection: skin ulceration, renal abscess, pus in the sinuses, a kidney stone blocking the urinary tract, infection due to an abortion, a perianal abscess, and infected wound, and so forth.

171—SEX

The Framingham Heart Study indicates that a nondiabetic nonsmoker in the general population has one chance in one million of having a heart attack during sexual activity and the one hour following. Patients with cardiovascular disease who pass a stress test have ten chances in one million. Individuals with angina have a higher risk: twenty-one chances in one million during sex and the two hours following.

This refers to the risk of nonfatal acute myocardial infarction. The risk of stroke or **sudden death is not exactly known, but it appears the risk is smaller than that for nonfatal myocardial infarction.**

In 1963, M. Ueno, a Japanese pathologist, published an article entitled "The So-called Coital Death." He studied the autopsies of 34 coital sudden-death victims during a four-year period. Interestingly, 25 of those deaths took place in hotel rooms, an additional 5 happened outside the home, and, in most cases, the deaths occurred during extramarital affairs. Moreover, all the victims had alcohol levels close to or within the range of intoxication, and their sexual partner was an average of 18 years younger.

In my book *Answering Your Questions About Heart Disease and Sex* **(Hatherleigh, 2007),** I relate the case of a sixty-five-year-old man who sustained an acute and massive myocardial infarction who left the intensive care unit just a few days after his admission to the hospital to have sex with a twenty-year-old girl. Was he crazy enough to do something like that? Yes, he was! Predictably, his funeral took place the same day.

Generally speaking, sex for the cardiac patient is a safe proposition, but it is important to identify those who are at high risk. This group of individuals should avoid sexual activity until their risk status changes for better and receive the medical advice to go back to intimacy.

High-Risk Patient

* Advanced chronic obstructive pulmonary disease (COPD)
* Certain types of congenital heart disease
* High-risk untreated cardiac arrhythmias
* Large thoracic or abdominal aortic aneurysms
* Severe cardiomyopathies

* Severe, uncorrected disease of the coronary arteries
* Recent acute myocardial infarction
* Recent congestive heart failure
* Recent stroke or TIA (transient ischemic attack)
* Severe carotid artery disease
* Severe pulmonary hypertension
* Severe valvular heart disease
* Uncontrolled hypertension
* Unstable angina
* Taking Viagra, Levitra, or Cialis when the blood pressure is too low
* Taking Viagra, Levitra, or Cialis with nitroglycerin or nitrates derivatives

The time for resumption of sexual activity should be advised by the health care practitioner, and in some cases, by the cardiologist. Usually, after an acute myocardial infarction, it may be resumed in 6-8 weeks, and those who undergo heart surgery, coronary bypass, or valve replacement, 4-6 weeks is usually appropriate. Again, this is a general idea, but your particular case must be evaluated in an individual, specific way, and medical instructions should be given according to your particular condition and not by what is "generally" done.

172—SLEEP APNEA

This disorder is underdiagnosed and undertreated.

Sleep apnea is a sleep disturbance where breathing pauses occur during sleep. This temporary absence of breathing is called apnea. An apnea event implies a minimum ten—second interval between breaths. The condition is usually diagnosed with an overnight sleep test called a polysomnogram (sleep study) usually done by a pulmonary specialist.

Sleep apnea is considered to be significant when the sleep apnea episodes occur five or more times per hour. There are three types of sleep apnea:

• Central
• Obstructive
• A combination of the above

Central sleep apnea (CSA) results from reduced respiratory effort due to a dysfunctional respiratory center in the nervous system. It is frequently seen in patients who suffer from congestive heart failure. Obstructive sleep apnea (OSA) is due to blockage of the upper respiratory tract. Occasionally, these two mechanisms are present in the same patient.

Obstructive sleep apnea (OSA) characteristically occurs in morbidly obese patients (weight excess of 100 lbs or more). The neck fatty tissue presses upon the upper respiratory tract, but other conditions may be responsible, e.g., large tonsils and adenoids, abnormal high-arched palates, genetic maxillo-facial abnormalities, nasal obstruction due to polyps, or deviated septum.

SYMPTOMS OF SLEEP-TROUBLED BREATHING

- Snoring
- Daytime sleepiness. Falling asleep during driving has caused accidents. It may also impair work performance due to fatigue
- Sleep interruptions at night
- Gasping or choking during sleep
- Morning headaches
- Poor memory
- Deficient concentration
- Fatigue
- Sexual dysfunction (reduced libido [sexual desire] and erectile failure)
- Irritability and moodiness
- Heartburn

Some of the above are only noted by relatives or a bed partner.

HOW IS OBSTRUCTIVE SLEEP APNEA DIAGNOSED

The best method is an overnight in-laboratory sleep study (polysomnography or PSG). Breathing patterns are evaluated, and samples of arterial oxygen, carbon dioxide concentration, and oxygen saturation are obtained. The patient is also monitored during the sleep by two electrode-encephalogram channels, eye movement recording channels, and one electromyogram channel, and measure of airflow at the nose and/or mouth.

TREATMENT OF OSA

- For obese patients, substantial weight loss is essential. At times, bariatric surgery (obesity surgery) is necessary
- Monitor intake of alcohol and tranquilizers
- Avoid smoking: airway inflammation makes a bad situation worse
- Supine position makes OSA worse. A tennis ball placed under the back may help some patients to avoid that position
- CPAP machine: this was introduced in 1981. It delivers positive pressure through the mouth or nose thereby preventing closure of the airway. The needed pressure varies from 4 to 20 cm of water. The problem with this machine is that some patients are noncompliant because they feel uncomfortable with it
- In special cases, mandibular and orthodontic devices are applied inside the mouth and displaced the mandible anteriorly, preventing the airway collapse

WHY OBSTRUCTIVE SLEEP APNEA MAY CAUSE A SUDDEN DEATH

An excess of sudden deaths during sleep between midnight and 6:00 a.m. in patients with OSA strongly suggests that this condition is capable of triggering lethal cardiac arrhythmias. Acceleration of the heartbeat may result from low oxygen concentration in the blood (hypoxemia); ventricular tachycardia and ventricular fibrillation may also occur during severe oxygen deficit, and also sympathetic nervous system stimulation, which is frequently associated with obstructive sleep apnea. In some instances, vagal stimulation leads to marked slowing of the heart rate or bradycardia and even a cardiac arrest.

The good news about obstructive sleep apnea is that it is treatable and preventable.

If you ever have an interview with a physician, a CPA, an attorney, or a corporate executive (it could be other professions too), and the individual is markedly obese and dozes off and falls asleep repeatedly and for a few seconds while you're talking to him, don't think he/she is intentionally neglecting you. Until proven otherwise, consider he or she is suffering from obstructive sleep apnea.

173—SHARK ATTACK

It was vacation time. I was eighteen, living in Argentina, and went to Mar del Plata, a charming town located about 500 miles from Buenos Aires. The Atlantic Ocean waters in this area are rather cold and choppy. I swam to a distance of about 300 feet from the beach.

All of a sudden, I saw a shark heading toward me. He was just a few feet away. It was a moment of intense suspense. There was no time to escape. There was no time to pray. When I saw him right in front of me, I instinctively kicked him with my foot. He made a quick rotation with his body and slapped my leg with his tail. It felt like a slap in my face. It was neat and powerful. I was scared. I began to swim back toward the beach, wondering if the shark was heading toward me for a second round.

I wanted to move as fast as a torpedo, but couldn't swim faster than a turtle. Luckily, the shark chose to do something else. When I touched the sand at the beach, I fell to the ground, exhausted.

People who saw me getting out of the water were screaming and alarmed. They told me that La Perla (that was the name of the beach) had been cancelled for swimmers due to an invasion of blue sharks. I had missed the posted warning signs.

THE BLUE SHARK

Blue sharks are ocean travelers. In New England they are among the largest in the world. The length of the blue shark may get over 9 ft, and their weight is between 300 and 450 lbs. They are fast swimmers and often form large all-male or all-female groups, which contain sharks of about the same size. No one knows why they do this. They are considered dangerous, and there have been attacks on people.

I was exalted with the realization that I had not been part of the shark's favorite menu.

Why did he decide not to bite me? Who knows? Perhaps he wasn't hungry. Almost surely he wasn't hungry!

I could never finish watching the movie *Jaws*. I'm sure you'll understand why!

WHY DOES THE SHARK ATTACK?

Some attacks seem to be purely inquisitive; others are probably due to "territorial rights" protection, need for feeding, involuntary interruption of the shark courtship activities, mistaken identity where water visibility is poor. Experts believe that most shark bites result from "prey identification mistakes": the shark is hunting a normal prey, whether fish, seal, or other food source, and mistakes a human for that prey. Large human recreational groups in the water also attract a shark attack.

TYPES OF ATTACK

Usually, the unprovoked shark attack involves a hit-and-run, bump-and-bite sequence.

Sneak attacks occur without warning.

The human bleeding from a shark bite may provoke further shark activity. Injuries are usually severe and occasionally fatal.

White sharks off the coast of California have been observed to kill their prey through a primary, violent bite, which results in the seal bleeding to death, after which the shark attacks.

Conversely, sharks in the Florida area are typically hunting fish, which they may consume in part or in whole in a single bite. These characteristics may explain why shark bites off the coast of California while much less frequent are more likely to result in death than are shark bites off the coast of Florida, which typically result in puncture wounds or lacerations.

BEST WAY TO AVOID A SHARK ATTACK

Play golf instead of swimming in the ocean!

RECOMMENDATIONS

Prevention

Lifeguard agencies should consult the United States Lifesaving Association Manual of Open Water Lifesaving and the International Shark Attack Web site (*http://www.flmnh.ufl.edu/fish/Sharks/ISAF/ISAF.htm*) for information and preventive actions that can be taken to reduce the chance of shark bites.

The best prevention is to have the awareness of what may invite a shark attack.

The following are general guidelines for swimming in areas inhabited by sharks:

- Swim, dive, or surf with other people—never alone. Avoid swimming in areas where sharks tend to congregate
- Avoid swimming in areas where sharks are usually found: between sandbars, near steep drop-offs, near channels, or at river mouths
- Don't swim in dirty or turbid water
- Avoid wearing shiny jewelry (this may simulate the scales of a prey fish)
- Avoid uneven tanning and contrasting
- Avoid bright-colored clothing
- Don't swim at dusk or at night
- Refrain from excessive splashing
- Keep pets and domestic animals out of the water. Their erratic movements call the sharks' attention
- Don't swim near sewage outfalls
- Avoid spreading blood or human wastes in the water
- If fishes start to behave erratically or congregate in large numbers, leave the area.
- If a shark is sighted in the area, leave the water as calmly and quickly as possible

Good luck with your next swimming!

174—SICKLE CELL CRISIS

Sickle cell disease (SCD) is the most common of hereditary blood disorders. It affects black Americans and black Africans. In the United States, 1 in 12 American blacks carry the gene of the disease. There are more than 50,000 persons seriously affected by this disorder.

In SCD many of the red blood cells have an abnormal shape, the sickle shape. These cells result from genetic mutations (changes) in the hemoglobin. These abnormal cells are stiff, distorted, and can't get through normally through small vessels and capillaries. The result is insufficient delivery of oxygen to various tissues and organs. This causes injuries, and sometimes, death.

When many of these abnormally shaped cells affect different areas of the body, the patient is said to have a sickle cell crisis.

A sickle cell crisis may involve the heart, blood, lungs, liver, bone, muscles, brain, spleen, penis, eyes, kidneys, and it may cause severe infections. The immune system is in disarray. This is due to the clogging of the spleen and its inability to serve its normal immunological defense duties.

WHAT CAN PROVOKE A SICKLE CELL CRISIS

- Fever
- Dehydration
- Infection
- Bleeding
- Hypoxia
- Cold exposure
- Drugs and alcohol
- Pregnancy and stress

CLINICAL MANIFESTATIONS

- Acute pain in the bone or bones
- Acute chest syndrome: shortness of breath, cough, and bloody sputum
- Abdominal pain. It is sudden and may become intolerable.
- Joint pain
- Kidney disease
- Eyes: retinal detachment
- Priapism (a constant erection). It happens in 40% of men affected by SCD
- Strokes: two-thirds of the strokes in people with SCD are children with average eight years of age.

TREATMENT

- If you have a sickle cell crisis, go the an ED fast
- In the hospital, treatment must deal with dehydration, infection, relief of pain, anemia (blood transfusions may be needed)

PREVENTION

- If you want to have children, get genetic counseling. If you received the gene from just one parent, you're a carrier. If you have sickle cell disease, you've received the genes from each of your parents
- Avoid low oxygen concentrations in your blood by not traveling in unpressurized airplanes or going to high altitudes
- Infants and young children with SCD have a high risk of bacterial infection and should receive penicillin every day until they are five years of age, and sometimes longer

WEB LINKS

- Sickle Cell Disease Association of America Inc.
- The Sickle Cell Information Center
- America Sickle Cell Anemia Association

175—SNAKE VENOM

Each year there are more than 45,000 snakebites in North America. There are many snake species. They are widely distributed throughout the world and various regions of the USA. **Some** of the poisonous snakes of the United States include **viper, cobra, rattlesnake, water moccasin, coral snake, copperhead.**

Each particular class of snake has its own colors, behavior, degree of aggressiveness, and toxin power. We can't go into details on snakes' characteristics. If you're going to travel to an area known to have snakes, for vacations or camping, or live in a region where snakes visit your backyard, and you, your children, and your pets play, rest, or have picnics, obtain more detailed information on the subject and become familiar with preventive measures and first aid management of a bite.

Some snakes are poisonous, others are very poisonous, and many of them are harmless. However, **if you don't know exactly the kind of snake that bit you, deal with it as an emergency and get to the nearest hospital emergency department (ED) immediately.**

Snakes bites can be deadly if not treated quickly. Children are at a higher risk for death or serious complications because of their smaller body size.

The right antivenom can save a person's life. If possible, call the emergency department by phone so the antivenom will be ready by the time the victim arrives there.

Symptoms depend on the type of snake: rattlesnake bites produce bleeding, shortness of breath, blurred vision, nausea and vomiting, paralysis, skin color changes, tissue damage, weak and rapid pulse, weakness, swelling.

Cottonmouth and copperhead bites include similar symptoms. Both of the above snakebites are painful and appear quickly.

Coral snakes bites may be painless at first, and significant symptoms may not develop for hours. Don't believe for a moment that if there is absence of pain at the bite's place and the bitten area looks fine, that everything is just fine. If untreated, coral snake bites can be deadly. Some of the symptoms include blurred vision, breathing difficulty, convulsions, headache, excessive salivation, swallowing difficulty, skin tissue damage, abdominal pain, paralysis, slurred speech, and shock.

If the area of the bite begins to swell and change color, the snake was probably poisonous.

FIRST AID

- Keep the person calm and provide reassurance that the wound can be treated
- Restrict movement
- Look for medical assistance fast. You may also call the National Poison Control Center (1-800-222-1222). The center can be called from anywhere in the United States. It is a national hotline number that will let you talk to experts. You'll get immediate advice and instructions. It is a free and confidential service
- Keep the affected area below heart level to reduce the flow of venom
- Remove any constricting items near the snake-bitten area because the bitten area may swell
- Immobilize the area loosely with a board, magazine, or other stiff material tied to the limb. Don't place it too tight. If you do that, you'll reduce the blood flow to the affected area, and you don't want to do that

- Do not try to suck out the venom by mouth. If you have a pump suction device such as that made by Sawyer, follow the manufacturer's directions
- Do not use a tourniquet. This will cut off blood flow, and the limb may be lost.
- Do not cut into a snakebite with a knife or a razor
- Do not give the person anything by mouth
- Do not give the victim stimulants or pain medications unless medically prescribed
- Avoid snakes altogether. If you see one, don't try to get closer to it, touch it, or catch it
- If the snake was killed and its head is being transported, be very careful because the decapitated head of the snake can still bite for up to an hour after it's dead (reflex action)
- Be careful with your hands and feet. Keep them away from areas where you cannot see well, like between rocks or in tall grass. Rattlesnakes like to rest in these areas

PREVENTION

- Avoid areas where snakes may be hiding, such as under rocks and logs
- Do not pick up or play with any snake
- If you do hiking, buy a snake bit kit, which is available in hiking supply stores.
- Never provoke a snake. Bites often occur from such behavior
- Tap ahead of you with a walking stick before stepping on an area where you can't see your feet. If the snake notices you're coming, it'll try to avoid you. Give the snake enough warning time
- When hiking or walking in an area known to have snakes, wear long pants and boots
- There are methods being sold to repel snakes, such as the Snake-A-Way repellent, naphthalene, a volatile product that vaporizes and creates an immediate interference that represses the snake's sensory system, scares it, and leads to its retreat

There's also a Sentinel electronic snake repeller that emits a pulsing vibration, which the snake picks up through sensors throughout its body. **The snake perceives a danger zone and evacuates the area. It is solar powered for economy and has low maintenance cost. It contains a solar panel and power cell that provide reliability for work continuously day and night.**

Each unit will protect 6,000 sq ft. The use of two units offer more protection than the use of one. To protect larger areas, multiple units are placed approximately 25 yd apart.

These methods have been reported to be effective most of the time but do not offer total guarantee of protection.

The rate of efficacy for the snake electronic repeller varies from 17% to 100%, but from fifteen different poisonous species tested, the Snake-a-Way product was reported to be effective, 91% to 100% of the times. This is a granular product that should be spread in a strip 10-30 centimeters apart, although generally, the wider the strip, the better.

176—SPLEEN RUPTURE

It was a trivial accident. The ten-year-old girl had been playing with her older brother who pushed her. She hit the corner of a kitchen table. Two days later, she suddenly developed acute abdominal pain and intense pallor. In the ED we quickly detected spleen rupture, and I myself pushed the stretcher to the operating room. She was bleeding internally, and her abdomen was filled up with blood. The spleen was removed and received several blood transfusions. She barely survived.

Another case involved another girl who fell off her bike and the steering hit her upper abdomen. That was enough to rupture the spleen.

What called my attention about these cases was the relatively trivial nature of the offending injury.

The spleen is an organ located in the left upper quadrant of the abdomen. It filters the blood by removing damaged or old blood cells and platelets. It also assists the immune system by destroying bacteria. So it does serve an useful function, but one can live a long life without this organ. In certain diseases, such as peculiar types of hemolytic anemias (the red blood cells become destroyed), the spleen is at times removed. A decreased resistance to infections occur following splenectomy (spleen surgical removal), so immunizations in these patients are very important.

177—STOPPING CLOPIDOGREL (PLAVIX) AFTER AN ACUTE CORONARY EVENT

Clopidogrel, commercially known as Plavix, is an extraordinarily useful medication regularly used for prevention of clots (thrombus) in the carotid arteries or the coronary arteries.

Current medical practice guidelines recommend clopidogrel therapy following an acute coronary syndrome for at least one month and as long as one year for patients treated medically or with barometal stents (BMS), and for at least one year for patients treated with drug-eluting stents.

A recent article in *Cardiology Review* (October 2008, vol. 25, no. 10) by P. Michael, MD, PhD and associates reported clot formation (thrombotic events) shortly after clopidogrel cessation.

In a national cohort of medically treated and also treated with coronary artery balloon and stents, the authors found a higher incidence of death and myocardial infarctions during the initial ninety-day period after clopidogrel cessation. The phenomenon seems to be related to a rebound effect of platelets activation associated with the drug's withdrawal.

Sometimes it just takes a few days or weeks after the drug was not taken to develop unstable cardiac symptoms again. **So be very careful and do not stop Plavix unless your doctor has a good reason to do it.**

178—SUDDEN DEATH IN ATHLETES

The Marathon Story that Changed the World

The year was 490 BC. The Persian and the Greeks (Athenians) were at war. The Persian had a powerful empire that extended from Asia to Egypt to what is now Turkey. The Greeks had scattered city-states, and their army was vastly outnumbered (4 to 1) by the Persians. But they made a very bold move: they launched a surprise attack, and hours later, over 6,000 Persian soldiers lay dead on the field while only 192 Athenians had been killed. Phidippides was one of the Greek fighters and a trained runner by profession. He was ordered to run to Athens to deliver the news of the victory after he had fought for several hours. He obviously pushed himself to the limit. He run twenty-six miles in about three hours, delivered the message, but dropped death as soon as he said, "We have won."

We don't know for sure if this was the first death by an intense physical effort by an athlete, but unquestionably, it's the most memorable. But why didn't Phidippides use a horse? It's been said that he had to cross mountains and rivers. So believe it or not, it was easier for him to run.

That was the marathon battle. The modern marathon race commemorates his tremendous feat. And there's a movie that relates this story, *The Giant of Marathon*, with Steeve Reeves.

In our days, young, superbly trained athletes at high school, college, or at a professional level, infrequently but repeatedly, suddenly hit the ground because of a cardiac arrest. Dr. Van Camp and associates described in 1995 160 cases of nontraumatic death in high school and college athletes between 1983 and 1993. Males outnumbered females 10:1. Other studies registered the same gender difference. A cardiac arrest in young females is very rare.

Sudden death occurs more commonly in males, and in the United States, football and basketball account for two-thirds of the athletes' sudden death. In other parts of the world, soccer is the number one sport associated with these quick demises.

Antonio Puerta, an internationally recognized soccer player, was playing for Sevilla FC, and on August 28, 2007, he died three days after having several cardiac arrests during a league game against Getafe. He had multiple organ failure and irreversible brain damage as a result had prolonged cardiac arrests. The cause of these arrests was a rare condition called arrhythmogenic right ventricular dysplasia (see section 100). Antonio's girlfriend was expecting their first child at the time of his death. He died on August 28, 2007, and his son was born a couple of months later. Sevilla FC retired Puerta's number 16 shirt, with the provision that should his son one day play for the club, he will have the exclusive option to use his father's shirt number.

Following Puerta's death, FIFA ordered the installation of resuscitation rooms in every stadium that hosted the South American World Cup qualifiers.

A tragedy like this is not unique. A few years ago, I was watching a soccer match between an African team and another one whose country of origin I don't remember. A soccer player collapsed and died in the field. Nobody helped him with CPR. Nobody knew what to do. Nobody touched him. It was a sad sight. The major contributor to sudden death from cardiovascular causes in athletes is hypertrophic cardiomyopathy (see section 88). The second most frequent cardiac cause of sudden death is congenital anomalies of coronary arteries (see section 55). Other causes include undiagnosed or unrecognized congenital heart disease and cardiomyopathies. A virus that presented as a flulike infection may invade the heart with little or no clinical recognition or awareness. Continued strenuous exercise during an acute myocarditis can lead to a cardiac arrest and sudden death. Some athletes have died suddenly due to selenium deficiency.

The estimated rates for nontraumatic sports death in high school and college athletes are 7.5 and 1.3 per million athletes per year in males and females, respectively.

Unfortunately, routine cardiovascular testing to prevent exercise-related sudden death in athletes is impractical and is not cost effective. Careful questioning about possible symptoms, such as dizziness, fainting, chest pains or discomfort, shortness of breath should not be neglected, and a physical examination may show a murmur that requires additional investigation.

179—SUDDEN DEATH IN THE MILITARY

The information that follows was obtained from an article published in the December 7, 2004 issue of *Annals of Internal Medicine* (vol. 141, 829-834) by R. E. Eckart, S. L. Scoville, and collaborators).

Sudden death occurs abruptly and unexpectedly without trauma or other obvious cause. Among 6.3 million military recruits, 126 nontraumatic sudden deaths occurred in recruits age 18-36 years from 1977 through 2001.

The researchers reviewed the military medical records and autopsy reports for all 126 recruits who died suddenly.

CONCLUSIONS

Death among military recruits is rare. It occurred in only 126 of 6.3 million recruits who entered basic training during this twenty-five-year period. Of the 126 deaths, 108 occurred during exercise. Fifty-one percent of the recruits who died (64 of 126) had a heart abnormality found at autopsy. The most common heart abnormalities involved abnormal origin of a coronary artery (61%), myocarditis (20%), and hypertrophic cardiomyopathy (13%).

More than one-third of sudden deaths remain unexplained after detailed medical investigation.

The duration of basic military training and the graduation requirements vary among the military services. In general, basic training may include basic rifle marksmanship, hand grenade, bayonet, hand-to-hand combat training, unarmed combat training, physical fitness tests (pushups, sit-ups, and a timed run, obstacle courses, live-fire exercises, foot marches up to 15 km, and field training exercises).

In athletes the most frequent cause of sudden death is hypertrophic cardiomyopathy. In this study involving military recruits, the most frequent culprit was congenital abnormalities involving a coronary artery (the left coronary artery taking off from the right sinus of valsalva). Myocarditis or inflammation of the heart muscle due to various viruses (echovirus, adenovirus, Coxsackie virus) was the second most frequent causes of sudden death. The third cause was hypertrophic cardiomyopathy. In any of the above, the mechanism of the sudden death was suspected to be due to an arrhythmia.

The recruit population is diverse: it includes women and various ethnic and socioeconomic groups. Pre-enlistment screening must carefully note if the applicant ever had previous cardiac symptoms of any kind or a significant family history of heart disease.

It is important to keep in mind that congenital anomalies of coronary arteries often give no symptoms, and the electrocardiogram and even treadmill or and nuclear cardiac stress tests may be negative. A CT scan or MRI may be required to detect the abnormality.

Dr. R. Eckart and associates (Harvard Medical School and Brigham and Women's Hospital) (Am J Cardiol, 2006 Jun 15; 97 (12):1756-8) studied the causes of sudden death in young female military recruits. From 1977 to 2001 approximately 852,000 women entered basic military training. During this period, there were 15 sudden deaths in female recruits, median age of nineteen years, 73% Afro American occurring at a median of 25 days after arrival for training. Sudden death with structurally normal hearts was the leading cause of death (8 recruits or 53%), and anomalous origin of a coronary artery was the second most frequent cause (2 recruits or 13% of the cases).

180—TETANUS

He was a family physician and lived with his ninety-year-old mother, a few yards from my house. I was a child and saw him often leaving his house with his medical bag to do house calls in the neighborhood. One day, his aging mother "became rigid and stiff," people in the little town commented. In two days she passed away. The cause of death was shocking to the curious neighbors: the doctor's mother died of **tetanus.**

Tetanus is a prolonged contraction of skeletal muscles. It results from the effects of a toxin produced by a bacteria called *Clostridium tetani* that penetrates the body through wound contamination, a skin cut, or a deep puncture. The jaw becomes contracted (lockjaw), the patient cannot swallow, and multiple muscles become spastic and stiff.

When I was working at Buenos Aires University, Department of Infectious Diseases, at the beginning of my medical career, we always had five to seven patients being treated for tetanus. The mortality rate was high. Many years passed since, and the mortality rate improved. In the United States, it is approximately 10%. The elderly and the unvaccinated and those who had a short incubation period carry the highest mortality.

The incubation period, namely the period between the wound and the presentation of tetanus symptoms, ranges from 3 to 21 days. The shorter that period is, the greater the likelihood of dying from this disease.

The most common presentation of tetanus is a generalized muscular contraction that goes from the head down. First, the patient contracts the jaw (trismus or lockjaw), then contracts the neck and back muscles and also the muscles of the extremities. These are painful contractions. The abdomen becomes rigid. The patient has swallowing difficulties, and the contracture of the respiratory muscles and the spasm of the larynx threaten the ventilation and respiratory function.

Spasms may occur frequently and last for several minutes. When the patient survives, these continue for about four weeks. Complete recovery may take months.

Neonatal tetanus occurs in newborn infants who suffer the disease because their mothers were never vaccinated. The infection occurs via an unhealed, infected umbilical stump. It is common in underdeveloped countries.

TREATMENT

- The wound's death and infected tissue must be surgically removed
- The patient should be treated with penicillin
- Those allergic to penicillin should receive one of these drugs: Clindamycin, metronidazole
- Passive immunization should be administered immediately with human antitetanospasmin immunoglobulin. If this is not available, use normal human immunoglobulin
- All victims must be vaccinated or given a booster shot.
- For mild tetanus, the following can be given:
  a) Tetanus immune globulin IV or IM
  b) Metronidazole IV for ten days
  c) Diazepam
- For severe tetanus, the following can be given:
  a) Human tetanus immunoglobulin is injected intrathecally (an intrathecal injection is given in the spinal canal, subarachnoid space)
  b) Tracheostomy and mechanical ventilation for a month
  c) Magnesium IV for muscular spasms
  d) Diazepam
  e) High caloric intake via gastric tube or intravenously. About 3,500-4,000 calories a day are necessary because of the energy spent by the frequent contraction of many muscles
  f) Other treatments for high fever, hypertension, or hypotension

PREVENTION = VACCINATION

Booster doses are given to adults every ten years or to any person with a puncture wound or a dirty wound. The booster does not prevent a potentially fatal outcome as it can take up to two weeks for tetanus antibodies to form.

Children under the age of seven usually get the DPT vaccine, which includes the vaccine against diphtheria, pertussis, and tetanus.

In the United States, tetanus affects about ninety persons annually, of which five of them die. Worldwide, tetanus remains a disaster. Three hundred thousand to 500,000 victims lose their lives every year.

181—VOODOO DEATH

Anthropologists and other people who have lived with primitive cultures in different parts of the world have testified that persons subjected to sorcery may be brought to death. This phenomenon has been observed in natives of South America, Africa, Australia, New Zealand, the islands of the Pacific, and Haiti.

Civilized people find it very difficult to comprehend this extraordinarily peculiar experience.

There are different ways of "executing" victims through voodoo. A popular "method" is that induced by a so-called medicine man in the Indian tribe who had the reputation of having supernatural powers. When he condemns a person to die, the degree of intimidation and fright is so extreme that the fear culminates in the victim's death. Sometimes, the death occurs in less than twenty-four hours. Other times, it takes a day or two, or even longer.

In Australia, scientists have stated that without doubt, from time to time, the natives die as a result of a bone being pointed at them. Particularly offensive in the tribal environment is failing to observe sacred tribal regulations. This is so firmly believed by all members of the natives' community that the selected victim and the victim him/herself that death is inevitable.

The big question here is whether a state of intense fear can end the life of a person. It is recognized that the perceived fear by the brain activates the sympathico-adrenal system that discharges an excess of adrenaline. This hormone causes a sudden increase in the blood pressure, constriction of the coronary arteries, and arrhythmias that may be lethal.

PART 7

SUDDEN INFANT DEATH

182—ABERRANT RIGHT SUBCLAVIAN ARTERY

This is a vascular anomaly, one of the so-called vascular ring abnormalities and has a congenital origin. The right subclavian artery arises from the aorta and normally reaches the right upper thorax. When the right subclavian artery has an abnormal origin, its course to the right upper thorax places the artery in front of the trachea and the esophagus. Sometimes, patients have no symptoms, but occasionally, the compression of the trachea causes acute bouts of shortness of breath, and the compression of the esophagus produces swallowing difficulties (dysphagia). In some infants, the trachea squeezing by the aberrant right subclavian artery has led to fatalities.

Diagnosis is made by simple barium swallow that shows a very characteristic esophageal indentation, and the diagnosis is confirmed by MRI and angiography. Correction requires surgery.

I once had an adult patient with this disorder whose dramatic symptoms of shortness of breath and swallowing difficulties had been missed since childhood (**Eduardo Chapunoff, MD, FACP, FACC, and Irwin Boruchow, MD, "Aberrant Right Subclavian Artery as a Cause of Respiratory Distress and Dysphagia in an Adult,"** *The Journal of the Florida Medical Association* **72:840-842 [Oct] 1985).**

183—CONGENITAL HEART DISEASE

Congenital heart defects are structural problems with the heart present at birth. They result from defective development soon after conception and often before the mother is aware that she's pregnant. Some defects are simple, such as "holes" communicating the atrial or ventricular chambers. Others are very severe malformations such as a single heart chamber or absence of valves, among many others.

If you already had a child with a congenital heart disorder or have a close relative with this problem, your chances for having a child with congenital heart disease are higher.

Out of 1,000 births, eight babies will have some kind of congenital heart defect. In America, about one million people have a congenital heart defect. Approximately 35,000 babies are born with a defect each year.

Most children with "simple" malformations survive to adulthood. Congenital heart defects, however, may be serious and fatal and are the most common birth defects during the first year of life.

The good news is that surgical management of some malformations has improved the mortality rate. In the 1960 and 1970s, it used to be around 30%, and nowadays, it has dropped to approximately 5%.

184—HYPERTHERMIA IN SUDDEN INFANT DEATH

Hyperthermia (abnormally high body temperature) could result from infection, often a respiratory infection although at times otherwise healthy babies may become overheated when they are covered or swaddled excessively or when they sleep prone. Heavy wrapping and excessive room heating also increase the risk of infant death. The human body has central nervous system thermo-regulatory centers. Sometimes, these are immature.

Infants lose much of their heat through the head and face, particularly when the rest of the body is covered. Prone sleeping significantly reduces the capacity for heat loss.

Infant and early childhood death caused by environmental hyperthermia (fatal heat stroke) typically occurs in vehicles or beds. The manner of death is either accidental or homicide.

Heatstroke occurs when a person's temperature exceeds 104 °F, and their thermo regulatory mechanisms are overwhelmed. A body temperature of 107 °F is considered lethal.

In patients less than two years of age undergoing cardiac surgery and requiring cardiopulmonary bypass, temperature elevations have been seen four to six hours after leaving the operating room. Use of intracardiac temperature monitoring has been suggested to avoid "cerebral hyperthermia."

The tragic death of a child left behind inside a car by the caregiver represents an example of an incredible degree of human stupidity. These deaths are totally and easily preventable. Over 300 infants and toddlers have died from hyperthermia in a hot car in the past decade in the United States alone. The hyperthermia occurs when a child (usually an infant or a toddler) is left unattended in a hot car and overheats beyond his or her body's ability to withstand it. Parents, older siblings, other relatives, nannies, family friends have all been guilty.

Never leave a child unattended in a vehicle, not even for a minute!

Always lock your car and ensure children do not have access to keys or remote entry devices.

How to Deal With It

- Obtain medical help immediately
- Turn down any heat source
- Remove excessive clothing
- Provide tepid water sponge bath
- Have them take acetaminophen 5-10 mg/kg per dose orally or rectally every four hours

185—HYPOTHERMIA

Hypothermia is low body temperature (an axillary or abdominal skin temperature below 35 °C).

Infants who are at a high risk of hypothermia are the following:

- Infants who are not dried well after birth
- Infants in a cold room or cool incubator
- Infants with low birth weight
- Infants lying near cold windows
- Infants who are starved

How do hypothermic infants look like?

1. They are cold to touch
2. They are lethargic, flaccid, have a feeble cry, and feed poorly
3. Their hands and feet are usually blue or pale, but their tongue and cheeks are usually pink. Careful now: the pink cheeks may incorrectly suggest that the infant is fine
4. They have shallow, slow breathing movements
5. They are bleeding from the mouth, nose, or needle punctures

The most frequent cause of death in hypothermic infants is hypoglycemia.

Cold infants use lots of energy trying to warm up themselves. In the process, they use up all their energy stores, and this results in hypoglycemia.

HOW IS INFANT HYPOTHERMIA TREATED?

- The infant must be warmed in a closed incubator or warm room. The incubator temperature should be set at 37 °C until the skin temperature returns to normal. If these are not available, the infant should be placed against the mother's skin and wrapped with a blanket
- Hypoglycemia may occur during warming. Energy can be provided by oral or nasogastric milk or intravenous dextrose 10%
- Provide oxygen 30% by **head box**
- Call for help to transport the infant to a hospital
- Keep the infant warm during transport

186—NEONATAL HEMORRHAGE

Hemorrhage is massive, heavy, or uncontrollable bleeding. Bleeding into the brain is one of the potential complications of a premature birth.

187—FATAL ACUTE MYOCARDITIS

This is a condition where the heart muscle is attacked by an infectious agent, usually a virus. The most common viruses are influenza virus, adenovirus, and Coxsackie virus although viruses such as rubella, rubeola, and HIV may also be responsible. Most of the damage is attributed to an immune reaction rather than the virus itself.

There are no known risk factors for developing this condition. Mild cases may recover, and the symptoms are so mild that they go unrecognized. Others are not so fortunate and develop severe weakness, accelerated heart rate associated with normal body temperature, shortness of breath, palpitations, or leg edemas, all of these consistent with heart failure.

Some babies followed a fulminant course of myocarditis and die immediately.

188—RESPIRATORY DISTRESS SYNDROME—IMMATURE RESPIRATORY CONTROL FUNCTION

Scientists have identified a gene critical to lung maturation in newborns and the production of surfactant, which lines lung tissues and prevents the lungs from collapsing. RDS (respiratory distress syndrome) is a common cause of death in preterm infants. The Cincinnati Children's helped pioneer the clinical use of surfactants to improve lung function in premature babies.

The Cincinnati Children's Hospital Medical Center is one of the America's top three children's hospital for general pediatrics and is highly ranked for its expertise in respiratory diseases, cancer, and digestive diseases. The hospital is a national and international referral center for complex cases.

Additional information can be obtained at *www.cincinnatichildrens.org*.

189—FATTY ACIDS DISORDER

There are infants who inherited disorders of fatty acid oxidation associated with enzymatic defects. These may present as isolated cardiomyopathy, sudden death, progressive skeletal myopathy, or liver failure. An arrhythmia may be the presenting symptom. This may result from accumulation of intermediary metabolites of fatty acids as long-chain acylcarnitines.

Inborn errors of fatty acid oxidation should be considered in babies found to have runs of ventricular tachycardia or unexplained sudden death. Diagnosis can be easily ascertained by an acylcarnitine profile from blood spots on filter paper.

190—REYE'S SYNDROME

Reye's syndrome is a deadly disease and affects children and adults in an acute manner and characteristically swiftly follows a fatal course. A life may be lost in a few days. The cause of it is unknown, but there has been an observed link between the use of aspirin and other salicylate-containing medications.

This disorder affects every organ of the human body, but the liver and the brain are particular targets. It is more frequently observed during January, February, and March when influenza is most common, but in reality, it also happens in the remaining months of the year. **When an epidemic of chicken pox or flu strikes, more cases of Reye's syndrome are seen. The disease is not contagious.**

The disease usually begins when a person is recovering from a viral illness. The liver quickly becomes fatty, and the pressure inside the brain increases. **It is important to diagnose and treat it as speedily as possible. When unrecognized or treatment starts too late, death is common in just a few days.** The treatment is supportive although no specific drug has been discovered to cure it.

SYMPTOMS

- Persistent vomiting
- Intense fatigue
- Drowsiness, confusion, disorientation
- Personality changes
- Aggressive and irrational behavior
- Delirium, convulsions, coma

CAREFUL ABOUT MAKING THE CORRECT DIAGNOSIS ON TIME

Doctors and medical staff who have not seen previous cases of Reye's syndrome may miss the diagnosis when the patient arrives at the emergency department. The characteristic protracted vomiting may be replaced in an infant with diarrhea.

The condition may mimic encephalitis, meningitis, drug overdose, poisoning, diabetes, or a psychiatric illness.

Although Reye's has been associated with use of aspirin and salicylates, the disease may occur without the ingestion of these medications.

The National Reye's Syndrome Foundation (it was founded in 1974), the U.S. Surgeon General, the Food and Drug Administration, and Centers for Disease Control and Prevention recommend that aspirin and a combination of products containing aspirin not be given to children or teenagers who are suffering from influenzalike illnesses and chicken pox.

National Reye's Syndrome Foundation Inc. e-mail: *nrsf@reyessyndrome.org* telephone: 1-419-924-9000

191—SUDDEN INFANT DEATH SYNDROME (SIDS)

SIDS is the leading cause of death among infants who are one month to one year old. Two thousand five hundred infants lose their lives each year in the United States. Most deaths due to SIDS occur between two and four months of age.

The prospect of losing a baby to this unpredictable and tragic event is frightening, to say the least. It appears suddenly and unexpectedly. You can only imagine what it means to the child's parents to wake up in the morning and see a dead baby who was, just a few hours prior, perfectly healthy.

What looks like SIDS probably is, but other conditions must be ruled out, such as a medical condition that parents' and the baby's pediatrician were not aware of, such as child abuse, an accident, or a metabolic or cardiac condition.

The incidence of SIDS increases in cold weather. Native American infants are three times more likely to die of SIDS than Caucasian infants. African American infants are twice as likely to run the same course. More boys than girls are victims of SIDS. It's been observed that there are also associated factors:

- Smoking, drinking, or drug use during pregnancy
- Deficient prenatal care
- Prematurity
- Low birth weight
- Mothers younger than twenty
- Smoke exposure after birth

- Excessive sleepwear and bedding
- Stomach sleeping

Stomach Sleeping

The very first thing you have to do is avoid placing the infant on his/her stomach to sleep. This position puts pressure on the child's jaw, narrows the airway, and impairs breathing.

Another mechanism that may cause an infant death with stomach sleeping is the risk of "rebreathing" his or her own exhaled air with a stuffed toy or a pillow close to the infant's face. The oxygen concentration of the air he or she breaths decreases, and the carbon dioxide concentration increases. This is defined as respiratory failure and may cause the demise.

Since the American Academy of Pediatrics recommended in 1992 that all healthy infants younger than one year of age be put to sleep on their backs, the rate of SIDS has dropped by over 50%. Despite of it all, still SIDS remains the leading cause of death in infants. So do not forget: **Put the baby to sleep on his/her back.**

Placing a baby in his/her side to sleep is not recommended. Why? Because there's a risk that the infant will roll over on to his/her belly while sleeping. Once the infant rolls over consistently (usually at age 4-7 months), it is OK to let the baby pick up a sleep position of his/her own.

Infants who die of SIDS may have an abnormality in an area of the brain called the arcuate nucleus that helps to control breathing and awakening during sleep. What this area does is to wake up the baby and make him or her cry. When the arcuate nucleus fails, the respiration is deficient, and the risk for SIDS is greater.

INFANT'S DANGEROUS ARRHYTHMIAS

Almost 10% of babies who die of SIDS have gene variations or mutations associated with potentially deadly heart rhythm disturbances. Drugs and implantable cardiac devices have been used to deal with this problem.

How to exactly identify this risk and prevent arrhythmia-related deaths during infancy hasn't been determined yet.

ADDITIONAL SUGGESTIONS TO REDUCE THE RISK OF SIDS

- Always place your baby on a firm mattress to sleep. Avoid pillows, **water bed**, or any soft surface
- To prevent "rebreathing," do not put blankets or pillows near the baby
- Make sure the room temperature where the baby sleeps is not too warm
- Never expose your baby to secondhand smoking
- Never smoke when you are pregnant. Infants of mothers who smoked during pregnancy are three times more likely to die of SIDS than those whose mothers were smoke free
- Make sure you have prenatal care
- Make sure your baby has regular checkups
- Breastfeed if possible. There's some evidence that breastfeeding decreases the incidence of SIDS
- If your baby has stomach reflux (GERDS), he/she needs to sleep in certain positions. Consult your doctor on this
- If the baby doesn't resist a pacifier, use it during the first year. This has been linked with lower risk of SIDS
- Do not sleep all night long with the baby. After sharing some moments in bed for nursing or comforting, return the baby to his/her crib. Parents inadvertently may roll over the baby and suffocate him/her

Parents and families who have experienced a SIDS death may consult the Sudden Infant Death Syndrome Alliance that provides counseling and support.

192—SUFFOCATION AND STRANGULATION AMONG INFANTS AND CHILDREN

Of course, it shouldn't happen. But reality prevails. Every year many infants and children die from strangulation and suffocation. These deaths can often be prevented. Parents and caregivers need to watch children closely and improve safety standards at home. The sleeping area is particularly dangerous.

The American Academy of Pediatrics, Centers for Disease Control and Prevention (CDC), and U.S. Consumer Product Safety Commission have provided the following safety tips to reduce the chances of suffocation and strangulation among infants and young children.

TO REDUCE THE CHANCES OF SUFFOCATION

At Bedtime

- Place babies to sleep on their backs on a firm, flat mattress
- Do not use pillows or heavy comforters in your baby's crib
- Make sure your baby's crib mattress is big enough for the crib. The space between the crib slats and the mattress should be smaller than the width of two adult fingers
- Never let your baby sleep in bed with you. Some babies have died when their breathing was blocked by pillows, bedding, and their parents
- Never let a baby sleep on a water bed. Fatalities occurred when the baby was trapped between the frame and the mattress

Around the House

- Keep plastics from shopping, garbage, and dry cleaning bags away from babies and children. Never use a plastic shipping bag or other plastic film as a mattress cover
- Choose a toy chest without a lid. If your child's toy chest has a lid, make sure it has a safety latch that stays open in any position. And make sure there are holes in the back or bottom of the chest to allow airflow, in case your child gets stuck inside
- Lock your car—including the trunk—when it's not in use. Keep the car keys away from children. Children have died after climbing into car trunks and becoming trapped
- **Always supervise children**

TO REDUCE THE CHANCES OF STRANGULATION

In the Crib

- Check with the U.S. Consumer Product Safety Commission before buying a new or secondhand crib to make sure it hasn't been recalled
- Make sure the slats on your crib are no more than 2 3/8 inches apart. This is specially important for secondhand cribs that are a few years old. If slides are wider than 2 3/8 inches apart, babies can slide through the slats and get strangled when their heads get stuck

- Do not use a crib with cutouts in the end panels or with corner posts more than 1/16 inch higher than the end panels. Strangulation can occur if a baby's clothing gets caught on a high corner post or if a baby's head gets caught in a cutout.
- Remove your baby's bib before bedtime or nap time
- Remove mobiles and crib gyms as soon as your baby is five months old or can push up on hands and knees

Around the House

- Pull drapery and miniblind cords out of children's reach and away from cribs. If the cords have a loop, cut the loop and attach separate tassels to avoid strangulation
- If your child has a bunk bed, check the guardrails on the top bunk. There should be only a very small space between the rail and the mattress or bed frame so your child's body cannot slide through
- Mini-hammocks, often used to store toys and stuffed animals, are also a hazard. Your child can get entangled in them
- Remove hood cords and drawstrings from your child's clothing. These cords can get caught in playground equipment or on crib parts and strangle your child
- Remove loose ribbon or strings on toys and stuffed animals. Never use a string or ribbon to tie a pacifier

In the United States, approximately fifty babies suffocate or strangle every year when they become trapped between broken crib parts or between parts of an older crib with an unsafe design.

Clothing and drawstrings also present a hazard for children, and there are several children who become strangled with fences, furniture, and playground equipment.

Resources

- American Academy of Pediatrics
  They have guidelines for parents
  www.medem.com

- U.S. Consumer Product Safety Commission
  They have information about toy safety, crib safety, and choking and
  strangulation risks
  www.cpsc.gov

- Juvenile Products Manufacturers Association
  They have a publication of JPMA that shows parents how to properly
  use products made for children
  www.jpma.org/public/safe-sound.html

- National Safety Council
  It offers a fact sheet on baby proofing your home *www.nsc.org/library/
  facts/babyprf.htm*

PART 8

SUDDEN DEATH IN PREGNANCY/ POSTPARTUM

193—ACUTE FATTY LIVER OF PREGNANCY (AFLP)

This is a rare but serious condition that appears during pregnancy in which there is an excessive accumulation of fat in the liver. Normal deposits of fat in the liver occur constantly (triglycerides and fatty acids). When these get into the liver in excessive amounts, liver damage takes place.

The cause of this disease is unknown. Risks are very high for the mother and fetus. It is life threatening and acts quickly. The mother has liver and kidney failure, hemorrhages in different parts of the body, and sepsis (severe infection in the blood). It usually begins in the third trimester of pregnancy, and it presents with nausea, vomiting, fatigue, headache, mental confusion, and jaundice (yellow coloring of skin and eyes).

The diagnosis is established by liver biopsy, taking a sample of liver tissue for examination under a microscope. A long needle is used to do it. This is not always possible in the pregnant woman. Ultrasound and CT scan that uses computer technology and produces cross-sectional slices of the liver may be used for diagnosis too.

The vital aspect of this condition's treatment is to deliver the baby as quickly as possible. Most cases react favorably.

194—ACUTE MYOCARDIAL INFARCTION AND CARDIOPULMONARY RESUSCITATION

This tends to occur in women who are older than thirty-three years of age who had several previous pregnancies. It generally happens during the last trimester of pregnancy and in the post partum period, from twenty-four hours to three months after delivery.

Studies in 125 patients have reported a maternal death rate of 21%. The demise usually takes place during the acute myocardial infarction, within two weeks of it, and it is commonly related to labor and delivery.

Most fetal deaths are associated with maternal deaths. Disease of the coronary arteries was found in 43% of patients and normal coronary arteries in 29%. The rest of the cases showed coronary arteries blocked by a clot (21%) or dissection (16%).

So although an acute myocardial infarction during pregnancy is a rare condition, it is a very serious and risky one, not only for the mother but for the fetus as well. If the mother survives, the fetus usually survives. The mortality rate of acute myocardial infarction related to pregnancy was shown to be 21%.

POSSIBLE CONTRIBUTING FACTORS

Some of the acute myocardial infarctions of pregnancy or those that occur during the postpartum are associated with a family history of coronary artery disease, low levels of "good" cholesterol (high-density lipoprotein), high levels of "bad" cholesterol (low-density lipoprotein), diabetes mellitus, smoking, or previous use of oral contraceptives.

Other contributing factors include clot formation inside a coronary artery (thrombosis), coronary artery spasm, collagen vascular disease, coronary artery dissection, cocaine use, aortic valvular disease, sickle cell disease, profound alterations in the coagulation process including platelet malfunction with tendency to clot formation, and marked changes in blood volume and heart rate that characterize the state of pregnancy.

DIAGNOSIS

Early recognition of an acute myocardial infarction during pregnancy does not happen easily. The reason is the low level of suspicion. Therefore, when there are suspicious chest discomforts, an electrocardiogram must be obtained immediately. Nuclear cardiac stress tests and cardiac catheterization deliver some radiation that could be harmful to the baby, and therefore, these must only be used when absolutely necessary. Termination of pregnancy is not generally recommended for fetal doses of radiation less than 0.05 Gy but may be considered when the dose exceeds that amount.

TREATMENT

The presence of the baby introduces important variables and limitations. The use of clot-dissolving agents (thrombolytics) is generally considered dangerous due to maternal hemorrhage and fetal loss, but in selected cases, it is not totally out of the question.

Nitrates can be used but with great care to avoid the mother's drop in blood pressure. Diuretics for heart failure should also be used carefully for the same reason.

All in all, some of the treatments provided for an acute myocardial infarction in a pregnant woman have significant limitations and precautions as compared with women who are not pregnant. The management of this condition is highly complex, and details go beyond the scope of this book. The patient must be treated in the intensive care unit, and anesthesiology and obstetric services need to be available at all times.

LABOR

To allow healing of the myocardial infarction, delivery should ideally be postponed for two to three weeks. Whether the delivery is done by C section or via vagina, both methods have advantages and disadvantages, and the cardiologist and obstetrician will have to make that delicate choice.

ISSUES RELATED TO CARDIOPULMONARY RESUSCITATION (CPR) DURING PREGNANCY

The fetus becomes viable at about the twenty-fourth week of pregnancy. Up until then, the treatment is guided almost exclusively by maternal considerations. Later, fetal safety becomes a serious issue too.

CPR in a pregnant woman has inconveniencies of its own: the distended abdomen makes the thorax less compressible and that may contribute to lower output of blood during chest compressions. Because of the pregnancy, the diaphragm muscle—the muscle that separates the thoracic and the abdominal cavities—is more elevated than normal, and by pushing the lungs up, it restricts the airflow.

The fetoplacental metabolism demands increase oxygen consumption. To increase the venous return to the heart, which is compromised because the pregnant uterus compresses the inferior vena cava, a pillow should be placed under the flank of the right abdomen and hip to displace to uterus to the left side. The person doing the CPR may use his or her own thighs while kneeling on the floor to serve the wedge purpose of a pillow.

Early evacuation of the uterus by bedside cesarean section results in recovery. Cesarean section after the thirty-second week of pregnancy should be considered if standard cardiopulmonary resuscitation is ineffective.

Survival of the infant has been directly proportional to the time interval between the death of the mother and delivery. Delivery that takes place more than fifteen minutes after maternal death rarely produces a viable infant, and almost all surviving infants have some neurological damage. Surviving infants delivered within five minutes after maternal death were healthy. To maximize survival of the mother and baby, rapid cesarean section (within four to five minutes of cardiac arrest) has been advocated.

195—AMNIOTIC FLUID EMBOLIZATION (AFE)

This is an obstetric emergency. It is fortunately rare (one case per 8,000-30,000 pregnancies) but affects the same all races and with a similar incidence all over the world. This disease was first discovered in 1941 when Dr. Steiner and Luschbaugh did the autopsy of a woman who had died during labor and found fragments of hair and other fetal debris in the lungs, specifically in branches of the pulmonary artery.

Even today, an air of mystery surrounds this disease. Initially, it was thought that amniotic fluid and fetal cells enter the maternal circulation and travel to the mother's lungs. Another possibility in some cases is an anaphylactic, hypersensitivity reaction to material of fetal origin that create an acute allergic type of reaction.

The usual presentation of this disorder is an acute cardiac arrest or severe hemorrhage that has no clear source, seizure, shortness of breath, cough, fluid in the lungs (pulmonary edema), and altered mental status (confusion, agitation).

Nobody knows how to prevent this disease. About 40% of these patients suffer from various allergies. Risk factors for its development include multiple pregnancies, advanced maternal age, male fetus, and trauma.

TREATMENT

This is supportive: oxygen, CPR when necessary, blood transfusions for severe anemia, and platelet transfusion for markedly decreased platelet count, and other heroic measures such as hemodialysis with plasmapheresis have occasionally saved a life.

In mothers who do not respond to cardiopulmonary resuscitation, emergent cesarean is indicated.

196—CEREBRAL ANEURYSM RUPTURE

Among women of reproductive age, the incidence of stroke is increased severalfold by pregnancy. Intracranial hemorrhage during pregnancy, from an intracranial aneurysm or an arteriovenous malformation, is a very serious complication that is responsible for 5-12% of all maternal deaths. The incidence of intracerebral bleeding due to a rupture cerebral artery aneurysm is about 1 in 1,000 pregnancies. Sometimes, patients complain of severe headaches; other times the initial presentation is a stroke.

The classic notion that a cerebral aneurysm in a pregnant woman tends to rupture during labor has not been confirmed. It's been reported that 90% of ruptures occurred during pregnancy and 8% during puerperium (the postpartum period).

Rupture of a cerebral aneurysm carries a high mortality. Pregnant women should be treated as nonpregnant patients and undergo operation when in good clinical condition. Some recover, but residual neurological damage may occur.

Those pregnant women with a ruptured aneurysm should have the aneurysm clipped as rapidly as possible. Once this is done, the pregnancy can be allowed to progress to term, and patient can be delivered vaginally if she is in good neurologic condition.

DSA (digital substraction angiogram) is the gold standard for the detection of cerebral aneurysms.

197—CONGENITAL HEART DISEASE AND PREGNANCY

The incidence of congenital heart disease (CHD) in the United States is estimated to be 0.5-0.8% or 32,000 new cases per year. Due to technological advances, 85% of children born with CHD now are surviving into adulthood. This has resulted in an increase in the number of females with CHD reaching childbearing age. CHD is now the predominant form of heart disease during pregnancy in developed countries.

CHD may have negative consequences for the pregnant woman: these include heart failure, arrhythmias, stroke, or death of the mother or fetus. During pregnancy the blood volume increases, and this imposes a burden on the heart. The amount of blood that the heart may be forced to eject is 80% greater than in the nonpregnant woman. Some heart congenital abnormalities are hazardous enough to contraindicate pregnancy to begin with, such as severe aortic or mitral stenosis, coarctation of the aorta, hypertrophic cardiomyopathy, and those with pulmonary hypertension. In contrast, leaking valves and lesions with interatrial or interventricular defects with no pulmonary hypertension are usually well tolerated.

Risk estimates and counseling of women with CHD ideally should be provided prior to conception. In general, vaginal delivery with a facilitated forceps delivery or vacuum extraction is the preferred route of delivery in patients with CHD. Cesarean section is indicated when obstetric reasons are present, in those patients on Coumadin, acute aortic dissection, Marfan syndrome with a dilated aortic root, and those with severe pulmonary hypertension and severe valvular obstructive lesions.

Many centers recommend endocarditis prophylaxis for women with CHD prior to delivery.

In general, pregnancy is well tolerated in patients with CHD. However, some patients have high-risk lesions, and pregnancy presents serious risks, including the risk of death. That is why risk stratification and preconception counseling are mandatory and should be done in all women with CHD of childbearing age.

Risks are estimated based upon the following:

- The heart anomaly
- Symptoms and functional capacity of the mother
- Necessity of having to surgically correct the heart abnormality prior to conception
- Additional factors that may complicate a pregnancy, such as a prosthetic valve, chronic anticoagulation, arrhythmias, or the use of an ACE inhibitor that may have adverse effects on the fetus
- The mother's ability to take care of the child
- The risk of the baby to inherit a serious congenital heart disease

198—HELLP SYNDROME

This is a rare but serious disorder. It can start abruptly, most often in the last three months of pregnancy or soon after delivery. HELLP stands for hemolysis (destruction of red blood cells), elevated liver enzymes levels, and a low platelet count.

The cause of this illness remains a mystery, and there's no way of predicting who is going to get it. There seems to be a prevalence of this disease in white women, older than twenty-five years of age, and those who had previous children.

HEELP symptoms include easy fatigability, abdominal pain, headaches, nausea and vomiting, swelling of face and hands, or bleeding from the gums or other places. Sometimes there's a blood pressure elevation. Most of the patients affected by this disease had hypertension before they became pregnant. When this illness turns ugly, it may be fatal. This is, though, a rare occurrence.

TREATMENT

The most important treatment of HEELP is to deliver the baby, and this might need to be done before the due delivery date. Sometimes it is possible to wait a few days. You may be prescribed steroids to help you and the baby, or blood transfusions if you bleed significantly. The usual response for the mother after delivering the baby is improvement. This becomes evident in a couple of days.

HOW TO PREVENT HELLP

There's no known way to do it. Your best bet is to have regular checkups by your obstetrician during prenatal visits.

Women who had HEELP once are more likely to experience it again during the next pregnancy, but the illness is usually less severe the second time.

PERIPARTUM CARDIOMYOPATHY (please see section 78)

199—PREECLAMPSIA

This disorder most often appears after the twentieth week of pregnancy. It presents with high blood pressure and spilling of protein in the urine. Edema may be added to this combination, but it is not necessary to establish the diagnosis of preeclampsia.

Eclampsia is the above-plus seizure activity.

The hypertension component of the disease is said to exist when the systolic blood pressure is greater than 140 mmHg or the diastolic blood pressure is greater than 90 mmHg when these numbers are recorded two times at least six hours apart, and in a woman who is known to have had normal blood pressure prior to pregnancy.

Protein in the urine (proteinuria) is present when the urinary protein concentration is greater than 300 mg during a twenty-four-hour period. If such test is not possible, then a concentration of at least 30 mg/dL in at least two random urine specimens collected six hours apart may be used.

Preeclampsia may be mild or severe. Recordings greater than 160 mmHg systolic or 110 mmHg diastolic associated with significant proteinuria classify the disorder as severe. Sometimes, there's associated heart failure, abdominal pain, liver function abnormalities, low platelet count, seizures, visual disturbances. The cause of this condition is not known. Preeclampsia occurs in about 7% of all pregnancies. The rate of eclampsia is 0.05%.

Preeclampsia is the second leading cause of maternal mortality, accounting for 12-18% of pregnancy-related deaths. Black women have twice the risk of preeclampsia compared to white women. Younger women have three times the risk of developing preeclampsia as older women.

Treatment must be carried out in a hospital. Mild cases can be treated with antihypertensive medications and drugs to prevent convulsions.

Failure of medical management demands vaginal delivery. If there are signs of maternal or fetal deterioration, emergent cesarean section is required. The only definitive treatment for preeclampsia is delivery of the fetus and placenta.

200—PULMONARY EMBOLISM (POSTPARTUM)

Venous thromboembolism is the release of lower extremity clots that travel north through the venous system to reach the heart, entering the right atrium, passing to the right ventricle, and from this cavity to the lung through the pulmonary artery.

It is a leading cause of maternal mortality and has been reported to occur in 0.5-3.0 of 1,000 pregnancies. Pregnancy increases the risk of venous thromboembolism by a factor of 5 over that of a nonpregnant woman of similar age. Predisposing factors are prolonged bed rest, pregnancy-related increased coagulability of the blood, decreased fibrinolytic activity (this means impaired body capacity to dissolve clots), and familial predisposition.

The usually recommended diagnostic test is the helical CT scan, which is not only safe during pregnancy but also accurate. Accuracy in the diagnosis of this disease is critical because there is a substantial risk for the mother and fetus. The recommended treatment for DVT (deep venous thrombosis) and PE (pulmonary embolization) during pregnancy is intravenous heparin for five to ten days followed by subcutaneously administered heparin for the remainder of the pregnancy.

The well-known anticoagulant warfarin (administered orally) is considered dangerous to the fetus so it is never used during pregnancy. For postpartum it should be used in combination with heparin initially followed by administration of warfarin alone for at least three months. Prophylactic programs of anticoagulation should be implemented in subsequent pregnancies.

The average fetal radiation dose with helical CT is less than with the V-P (ventilation perfusion) lung scan. Pregnancy should not preclude the use of helical CT for the diagnosis of pulmonary embolism.

201—SEPSIS DURING PREGNANCY

The incidence of maternal mortality related to sepsis has decreased during the past two decades due to the availability of a wide variety of antibiotics and the technological advances in critical care. Still, when sepsis occurs in the pregnant woman, it may be fatal. The most common infections are chorioamnionitis (infection of the amniotic fluid), endomyometritis (infection of the inner layer of the uterus that usually follows delivery by cesarean), septic abortion, pneumonia, and pyelonephritis (severe kidney infection).

Early recognition of sepsis is crucial to prevent septic shock and death. Usually, these infections in the pregnant woman respond to broad-spectrum antibiotics.

EPILOGUE

In the course of this book, I discussed multiple causes of sudden or rapid death in a brief manner. I dealt with many of them but, by no means, all of them. Terrorism wasn't discussed, and one can certainly die suddenly or rapidly because of it. Homicides were also avoided except for a rare mention. Accidents were briefly dealt with, and this was also part of these calculated omissions. Rare medical conditions of genetic origin were avoided too. The same applies to various poisons. Dealing with them would have meant writing an encyclopedia, but this was not my intention when I planned this work.

More than anything else, I wanted you to become aware about many potential dangers you or people you care about might face in a lifetime. Although I often cited methods of treatments, the main purpose of this journey dealing with deadly sudden and rapid experiences is to remind you about their existence, how dangerous they are, how to prevent them, and in many instances, the basics on how to deal with them.

I insist on this particular point: never use this book to treat yourself or someone else. The science and art of medicine is complex, and you've got to spend years of your life not only to become a health professional, but to be a very good one.

Those who die suddenly or rapidly—as well as those who die slowly—are not coming back. Their departure from this world leaves behind not only a sadness difficult to overcome, but also the extraordinary experience of their ordeal. We should be ready to learn from it. I'm sure that those who died suddenly or rapidly would gladly tell us: *"Be careful, look what happened to me. I died in the wrong place and at the wrong time. If I just had another chance! . . . Had I read and learned more about the way I died, I'm certain I could have lived longer!"*

I can't imagine any reasonable individual who would not be interested in preventing his/her own death or the death of a beloved person. And this applies to people of any age, race, nationality, educational level, socioeconomic status, religion, and profession.

It is my deep desire and hope that you'll find this guide useful.

Eduardo Chapunoff

RESOURCES

AGING

National Institute on Aging
Building 31 Room 5C27
31 Center Ddrive, MSC 2292
Bethesda, MD 20292

—*—

National Council on Aging
409 Third Street SW, Suite 200
Washington DC 20024
1-800-424-9046

—*—

ALCOHOL

1-800-ALCOHOL

This hotline is available twenty-four hours a day, seven days a week. They offer counseling and assistance in finding local treatment centers.

—*—

Alcoholic Anonymous Inc.
General Service Office
PO Box 459
Grand Central Station
New York, NY 10163
212-870-3400

—*—

Alcohol and Drug Abuse hotline 1-800-454-8966
Children of the Night
1-800-551-1300

—*—

CANCER

American Cancer Society
National Office
1599 Clifton Road NE
Atlanta, GA 30329

—*—

CARDIOVASCULAR HEALTH

American Heart Association
National Center
7272 Greenview Ave
Dallas, TX 75231-4596
1-800-242-8721

—*—

American Red Cross National Headquarters
2025 E. Street NW
Washington DC 20006
202-303-5000

—*—

National Heart, Lung, and Blood Institute
Information Center
PO Box 30105
Bethesda, MD 20824-0105

—*—

Sudden Arrhythmia Death Syndrome Foundation
PO Box 58767
Salt Lake City, UT 84158

—*—

National Institute of Neurological Disorders and Stroke
NINDS Information Service
Building 31, Room 8, A06
Bethesda, MD 20892
301-496-5751

—*—

National Stroke Association
300 East Hampden Ave., Suite 200
Englewood, CO 80110-2622

—*—

American Stroke Association
1-888-478-7653

—*—

DIABETES

American Diabetes Association, Inc.
1660 Duke Street
Alexandria, VA 22314
1-800-232-3472

—*—

National Diabetes Information Clearinghouse
One Information Way
Bethesda, MD 20892-3560

—*—

DRUGS

National Institute on Drug Abuse
1-800-662-4357

—*—

Narcotics Anonymous
www.na.org

—*—

GENERAL HEALTH SERVICES AND INFORMATION

National Library of Medicine
8600 Rockville Pike
Bethesda, MD 20894
1-800-272-4787

—*—

MENTAL HEALTH ORGANIZATIONS

The National Mental Health Association
www.nmha.org

—*—

Mental Health Net-Self Help Source Book mentalhelp.net/selfhelp

If you have suicidal thoughts:

- Dial 911
- Dial 1-800-272-TALK
- Go to a hospital emergency room immediately

  The yellow pages usually list the local suicide prevention hotline or crisis center. The Trevor Project 866-488-7386 aims at gay and questioning youth (toll-free suicide prevention hotline).

  Girls and Boys Town Crisis Line, twenty-four hours a day, every day 1-800-448-3000

MORBID OBESITY

Morbid Obesity and the Struggle for Survival (Book-2007)
Eduardo Chapunoff, MD, FACP, FACC
Publisher: iUniverse

**

Morbid Obesity: Will You Allow it to Kill You? (2010)
Eduardo Chapunoff, MD, FACP, FACC
Publisher: Xlibris

POISONS

National Capital Poison Center
1-800-222-1222

American Association of Poison Control Center
www.aa[cc/org/DNN/

SEX AND HEART DISEASE

Answering Your Questions About Heart Disease and Sex (Book-2007)
Eduardo Chapunoff, MD, FACP, FACC
Publisher: Hatherleigh, NY
Distributor: Random House

SICKLE CELL DISEASE

Sickle Cell Disease Association of America Inc.
231 East Baltimore St. Suite 800
Baltimore, Maryland 21202
scdaa@sicklecelldisease.or

SCUBA DIVING Information
Divers Alert Network
www.diversalertnetwork.org

—*—

National Oceanic and Atmospheric Administration
www.noaa.gov

—*—

Doc's Diving Medicine (underwater medicine information)
http://faculty.washington.edu/ekay

—*—

GLOSSARY

A

Abdominal Aortic Aneurysm—AAA. Focal dilatation of the abdominal aorta

Ablation. Elimination of a localized area of cardiac muscle responsible for causing severe tachycardia. One common ablation technique is "radiofrequency ablation". It is done by introducing wires (catheters) inside the cardiac chambers through the groin blood vessels

Ace-inhibitor. A drug used to treat hypertension and heart failure

Acute fatty liver of pregnancy. Rare but serious disorder. The liver accumulate excessive fat during pregnancy. Treatment consists in delivering the baby as quickly as possible

Acute rheumatic fever. An inflammatory disease that sometimes follows group A Streptococcal infection of the throat

Adrenal insufficiency. Disease caused by insufficient production of cortisone derivatives (steroids) in the circulating blood

Adrenaline. Also known as epinephrine. A hormone produced by the adrenal glands that increases the heart rate and relieves bronchial spasm

Advanced heart block. The electrical impulse of the upper chambers of the heart (atria) doesn't get transmitted to the lower chambers (ventricles). The heart rate drops down to 40 beats per minute, or less

Airway obstruction. Blockage of the airways. It may be at the level of the upper respiratory tract (larynx and trachea), or in the lungs (bronchi) where it is called COPD (chronic obstructive pulmonary disease)

Alcoholic cardiomyopathy. Weak and dilated cardiac chambers that result from the chronic alcoholism

Amyloidosis. A group of protein deposition diseases that causes disruption of normal function in multiple organs

Anabolic steroids. Substances that have been often used by athletes to heighten their performance and muscular mass. At times, they can be dangerous and affect the liver, heart, and other organs. Young athletes have developed premature coronary artery disease, myocardial infarctions, and strokes

Anaphylaxis. Acute generalized allergic reaction that requires emergency management

Aneurysm. Focal dilatation of an artery that results from weakness of the arterial wall

Angina—Also called Angina Pectoris. Pain or discomfort usually—but not always—located in the mid-anterior chest due to insufficient blood delivered to the heart muscle—usually due to obstruction of a coronary artery

Angiogram (angiography). X ray picture of arteries that have been injected with a radio-opaque substance that allows them to be seen and analyzed. If the coronary arteries are investigated, the test is called a coronary angiogram

Angioplasty. Treatment of an atherosclerotic plaque that severely narrows an artery, by the use of a wire (catheter) that has a balloon at its tip. This is positioned at the level of the blockage, and when it is inflated, it relieves the obstruction and restores blood flow

Anorexa Nervosa. Eating disorder. The patient has the perception of having excessive adiposity, when, in reality, he/she is extremely thin

Anticoagulant. Blood thinner. It prevents the formation of blood clots

Antracycline-induced cardiomyopathy. A weak and dilated heart that results from the use of the anticancer drug called antracycline

Aortic dissection. Circulating blood is propelled into the middle or outer layer of the aorta due to a tear that occurs in the inner layer of this artery

Aortic regurgitation. Aortic valve leakage due insufficient valve closure

Aortic stenosis. Narrowing of the aortic valve orifice

Appendicitis. Acute inflammation of the appendix

Arrhythmia. Any abnormal heart beat rhythm

Arrhythmogenic right ventricular dysplasia—ARVD. A right ventricular cardiomyopathy characterized by fatty replacement of the myocardium. Sometimes, it leads to serious arrhythmias. It can be treated with medications, ablation, or an intracardiac defibrillator

Arterial spasm. Constriction of an artery

Apnea. Airflow cessation for at least 10 seconds

Asphyxia. Severe oxygen deficiency in the body

Asymptomatic. Lack of symptoms

Asthma. A respiratory disease that causes bronchial spasms (constriction of the bronchial tubes), wheezing, coughing, chest tightness, and shortness of breath

Atheroma. Localized fatty material that forms a plaque inside an artery

Atherosclerosis. A process that primarily affects the inner layer of an artery and forms the atherosclerotic plaque

Atrial fibrillation. Irregular heart beat due to an abnormality of the atrial chambers

Atrium. One of the two small upper chambers of the heart

B

Bends. Damage that results from bubbles released in the bloodstream during scuba diving's too rapid ascent toward the surface that can cause a myocardial infarction, stroke, and/or leg paralysis

Beta-blocker. Drug used to treat angina pectoris, hypertension, heart failure, arrhythmias, familial tremor, and migraine headaches

Brugada syndrome. A condition diagnosed by typical abnormalities in the electrocardiogram that can be associated with life-threatening cardiac arrhythmias

C

Cardiac arrest. Cessation of the normal heart beating, that is replaced by a chaotic rhythm called "ventricular fibrillation" (VF), or a straight line, called "asystole"

Cardiac catheterization. A procedure that involves the insertion of a fine tube (catheter) into an artery, usually in the groin area, and passing the tube into the heart. It is done under local anesthesia. It evaluates the status of the heart function and valves, and it is usually used in conjunction with the coronary angiogram, which identifies obstruction of coronary arteries, their precise location and severity. It is often an indispensable tool in the diagnosis and treatment of heart disease

Cardiogenic shock. Advanced failure of the heart to produce a viable blood pressure in the circulatory system

Cardiomyopathy. A disease of the heart muscle that often results in deterioration of the heart's pumping ability

Cardiopulmonary resuscitation—CPR. Procedure to revive a person who sustained a cardio-pulmonary arrest

Cardioversion. A technique that applies an electrical shock to the chest in an attempt to correct a rhythm disturbance. Cardioversion can be also successful with the use of intravenous antiarrhythmic drugs

Cerebral aneurysm—"Berry" aneurysm. A focal dilatation of a cerebral artery

Cerebral hemorrhage. Bleeding inside the brain due to rupture of a cerebral artery

Cerebral infarction. Brain damage that results from the suppression of blood supply to an area of the brain due to a blocked cerebral artery

Cholesterol. One of many fatty substances that circulate in the blood and contributes to atherosclerosis

Circadian rhythms. The body's 24 hour-pattern that involves multiple processes of cyclical activity, such as sleep, hormones, blood pressure, and many others

Collateral circulation. Dormant vessels that dilate and become active and useful when there's a chronic and severe arterial obstruction. Their presence in the heart may prevent an acute myocardial infarction

Commotion Cordis. An often relatively trivial contusion in the chest that, unluckily, may affect the victim at a highly vulnerable electrical period of the heart beat, and cause a cardiac arrest

Conducting system. Bundles distributed throughout the heart muscle that carry the electrical impulse that will activate the heart and make it contract

Congestive heart failure. Fluid accumulation in the lungs and other tissues (liver, lower extremities) that results from a weak heart muscle

Coronary angiography. Films obtained from the coronary arteries when they are injected a contrast material for their visualization. It is part of the cardiac catheterization

Coronary artery disease. Symptoms and complications that result from coronary atherosclerosis

Coronary atherosclerosis. Plaques that contain cholesterol inside the coronary arteries

Coronary insufficiency. Symptoms or events that result from coronary artery disease

D

D.C. shock. Electrical current applied to the chest through pad electrodes to eliminate an arrhythmia

Deep venous thrombosis—DVT—Clot formed in a deep vein

Defibrillator. A machine or equipment that produces an electrical discharge aimed at the correction of ventricular tachycardia or ventricular fibrillation

Diastole. Each cardiac expansion and relaxation

Dyslipidemia. Abnormal blood lipid levels

Dyspnea. Breathing difficulty

E

Ejection Fraction. The % of blood ejected by the left ventricle. It reflects the contractile strength—or weakness—of the cardiac muscle

Encephalitis. Acute viral infection of the brain

Endocarditis. Infection of the heart valves

Erotic asphyxia. Mental disorder that seeks enhancement of sexual pleasure by self-induced asphyxia

Eutanasia. Medically-assisted death

H

HDL. High density lipoprotein, also called the "good cholesterol"

Heimlich Maneuver. Method that everybody should know to relieve an acute upper airway obstruction caused by a foreign body

Hemochromatosis. Excessive iron deposition in various organs, the heart included

Hemolytic anemia. Anemia that results from the rupture of many red blood cells

Holter monitor. A recording of the heart beat, usually for 24 hours for detection of cardiac arrythmias (Holter is the name of the engineer who created the method)

Hypercalcemia. Abnormally high serum calcium levels

Hyperkalemia. Abnormally high serum potassium levels

Hypersensitive carotid sinus. Severe slowing of the heart rate that follows compression of an area in the carotid arteries called "the carotid sinus". This severe bradycardia may follow manual compression of the carotid artery or may also result from certain motions of the neck

Hypertension. High blood pressure

Hypertensive cardiomyopathy. Heart disease that results from chronic arterial hypertension

Hypertensive cardiovascular disease. Cardiovascular disease that results from chronic or acute arterial hypertension

Hyperthermia. Above normal body temperature

Hyperthyrodism. Excessive production of thyroid hormone by a hyperfunctioning thyroid gland

Hypertrophic cardiomyopathy. Thick heart muscle

Hypertrophic obstructive cardiomyopathy. Thick heart muscle that blocks the exit of blood from the ventricle

Hypocalcemia. Low levels of serum calcium

Hypoglycemia. Abnormally low levels of blood glucose

Hypokalemia. Low levels of serum potassium

Hypomagnesemia. Low serum levels of magnesium

Hypotension. Low blood pressure

Hypothermia. Below normal body temperature

Hypothyroidism. Deficient production of thyroid hormone by the thyroid gland

I

Idiopathic dilated cardiomyopathy—IDC. Dilated and weakened heart muscle that may result from a virus, alcoholism, pregnancy, and other causes

Infarction. Damage to an organ that results from an occluded artery. It may happen in the brain, heart muscle (myocardium), spleen, and other organs

Ischemia. Deficient blood supply to an organ

L

Laryngeal spasm. Constriction of the larynx that may produce snoring-like noise and severe respiratory embarrassment

LDL. Low density lipoprotein, also called the "bad cholesterol"

Left atrial thrombus. Clot located inside the left atrium

Left ventricular aneurysm. Damaged heart muscle that resulted from an acute myocardial infarction and that bulges outwards when the rest of the heart muscle contracts inwardly. It may lead to arrhythmias and heart failure

Left ventricular pseudoaneurysm. It may look like a ventricular aneurysm, but it is not. This lesion results from a small perforation of the heart muscle that suffered a myocardial infarction. The blood drains into the pericardium and gives the appearance of a true aneurysm. A true aneurysm is scarred muscle. A pseudoaneurysm is an accumulation of blood

Left ventricular thrombus. Clot inside the left ventricle

Lipids. Collectively, the cholesterol and its fractions, HDL, LDL, triglycerides

Lipoproteins. The vehicles that cholesterol and other lipids fractions use for transport in the blood

Liver failure, acute, fulminant. Critical acute liver damage. Poisoning with acetaminophen with suicidal attempt is a frequent cause

M

Malignant hypertension due to general anesthesia. Infrequent but very important and difficult to control hypertension due to a general anesthetic

Meningitis. Acute infection of the membranes that cover the brain, usually produced by bacterias

Meningococcemia. Sepsis due to an abundance of germs called meningococci

Mitral regurgitation. Leakage of the mitral valve. It results from abnormalities affecting the mitral valve per se or the mitral valve apparatus, that includes the tissues that hold the valve to the ventricular wall, namely, the chorda tendinea and the papillary muscles

Mitral stenosis. Narrowing of the mitral valve. The blood moves from the left atrium to the left ventricle with difficulty. It may be due to old rheumatic fever, a congenitally abnormal valve, or occur in the elderly due to severe calcification of the mitral valve leaflets

Mitral valve prolapse (MVP). Some ballooning of the mitral valve leaflet (s) during each ventricular contraction, usually due to excessive or redundant valve tissue

Morbid obesity. A condition diagnosed when the patient carries 100 lbs or more of weight excess

Morbidity. Complications and disabilities of a disease

Murmur. Heart sound detected by the stethoscope that indicates that a valve is too narrowed (stenosis), or can not close properly (insufficiency or regurgitation

Muscular dystrophies. A group of genetic disorders, some of which are associated with heart failure and rhythm disturbances

Myocardial infarction. Heart damage that results from acute deprivation of blood to a portion of the heart muscle, usually resulting from a blocked coronary artery

Myxoma. The most frequent benign intracardiac tumor. In some intracardiac locations, it's capable of causing serious "mechanical" problems

N

Non-compaction cardiomyopathy. A recently described genetic disorder characterized by enlarged and loose trabeculae seen in the depths of the ventricle's muscle

Non-invasive procedure. Any diagnostic or treatment procedure in which no instrument enters the body

P

Pacemaker. Instrument that produces cardiac muscle stimulation when the patient's own beats fail to appear when needed

Pacemaker malfunction. The artificial pacemaker does not act properly. This can be resolved by high technology instruments at the bedside but sometimes, a reoperation is necessary

Pericardial tamponade. Dangerous blood or fluid accumulation inside the pericardial cavity

Pericarditis. Inflammation of the pericardium

Pericardium. Membrane that covers the heart. It has two layers and a small amount of fluid in between them

Peri-partum cardiomyopathy. A dilated and weakened heart that develops 3 months prior to delivery or shortly following it. The cause is unknown

Peritonitis. Acute, dangerous infection of the peritoneal cavity

Positional asphyxia. Inability of a person to breathe when he/she was restrained with the face down and was compressed his/her thorax

Pre-eclampsia. A disorder that most often appears during the 20th week of pregnancy. It presents with high blood pressure and spilling of protein in the urine. (Eclampsia is the same plus seizure activity)

Proarrhythmic drug. Any drug that causes an arrhythmia

Prosthetic cardiac valve. An artificial heart valve. It may be a mechanical or tissue valve

Prosthetic cardiac valve dysfunction. A malfunctioning prosthetic valve

Psychiatric polypharmacy. Use of multiple antipsychotic drugs in a single patient

Pulmonary embolization. Clots released by the veins—usually those of the lower extremities-that reach the lungs

Pulmonary hypertension. High pressure in the arterial territory of both lungs.

R

Radiation poisoning. Intentional use of radioactive material for criminal purposes

Radiation treatment complications. Unintentional but common complications that result from standard doses of radiation to cure cancer

Respiratory failure, acute. Severe, acute inability of the respiratory system to provide the human body with adequate oxygenation

Reye's Syndrome. It is a disease of unknown origin that affects children and adults, and typically follows a rapid fatal course. It usually appears during recovery from a viral illness. It has been observed a link between this disorder and the use of aspiring and other salicylate-containing medications

Rupture of chorda tendinea. Anatomical disruption of structures that holds the heart valves. It causes severe mitral valve regurgitation

S

Sepsis. Abundance of bacterias in the bloodstream

Sick Sinus Syndrome (SSS). Failure of the Sinus Node to produce a normal heart beat. This results in severe slowing of the heart rate (bradycardia)

Sickle Cell Crisis. An acute destruction of abnormal red blood cells, called sickle cells, that affects multiple organs

Silent heart attack. A myocardial infarction that occurred without any symptoms. It happens in approximately 15% of all heart attacks.

Sinus Node. This is the natural pacemaker of the heart located in the right atrium. It measures 20 mm by 5 mm and generates the electrical impulse that is transmitted to the rest of the heart's conducting or electrical system

Sleep apnea. Sleep disturbance where breathing pauses occur during sleep

Sleep Death. Lethal arrhythmias that occur in patients younger than 45. Most affected are of Asian origin

Splanchnic artery aneurysm. Usually unsuspected aneurysms of some abdominal arteries, e.g., spleen, intestines, that may cause abdominal pains. Sometimes, these burst

Spleen rupture. It sometimes happens during relatively minor accidents, such as falling against the edge of a table, or falling off a bike. Always needs immediate surgical treatment

Standstill. Total cessation of the heart beat. The ECG only shows a straight line

Status Epilepticus. Persistent, recurrent attacks of epilepsy that are difficult to control

Stent. A device make of expandable metal mesh that is placed at the site of a narrowed artery after this was dilated by a little balloon located at the tip of a catheter. The stent is then expanded to keep the artery open

Stress test. Method to detect deficient blood supply to the cardiac muscle. It can be done by exercising the patient under electrocardiographic monitoring, using echocardiogram to detect ventricular wall motion abnormalities, or nuclear material injections for identification of cardiac muscle regions that are not well perfused (not receiving the appropriate blood supply

Stroke. Damage that results from the blockage of a cerebral or carotid artery, or a cerebral hemorrhage

Sudden Infant Death Syndrome—SIDS. The leading cause of death among infants who are 1 month to 1 year old

Syncope. Acute total loss of consciousnes

Systole. Each cardiac contraction

T

Thyroid Storm. An acute, life-threatening condition due to an uncontrolled release of thyroid hormone into the bloodstream

TIA—Transient Ischemic Attack. Temporary deficiency of blood supply in the brain tissue that lasts from minutes to several hours, and does not produce permanent damage. The stroke does

Thrombus. Intra-arterial or intravenous clot

Triglycerides. A group of blood lipids that is associated with cardiovascular disease, when the blood levels are high

U

Unrecognized myocardial infarction. A myocardial infarction that occurred with symptoms different from those seen during a typical heart attack. Instead of chest pain, the pain may be located in the ear lobe, abdomen, elbow, between the shoulder blades, or cause profound weakness, shortness of breath, or fainting. 33% of all myocardial infarctions go unrecognized by the patient, the doctor, or both

V

Vasoconstriction. Reversible narrowing of veins or arteries

Vasodilatation. Reversible widening of veins or arteries

Vasospasm. Constriction of a vein or an artery

Venous insufficiency. Disease of the veins, which can not collect the blood properly from the lower extremities

Ventricular ectopic or premature beats. Extra beats. Their meaning and importance require a clinical evaluation

Ventricular tachycardia. Abnormal fast rhythm that originates in the ventricles

Ventricular fibrillation. Chaotic cardiac rhythm that leads to death unless it is quickly reversed

W

Wolf-Parkinson-White syndrome. A condition that presents peculiar ECG features. It results from presence of a bypass tract that delivers the normally produced electrical discharge into an abnormal tract instead of the normal atrio-ventricular conduction. The condition may cause no symptoms, or tachycardia episodes of varying severity

INDEX

A

AAA (ABDOMINAL AORTIC
ANEURYSM), 30–32, 42, 179,
182, 203, 222, 247, 287, 337
abdominal wounds, 173
ablation, 145, 158, 162, 168, 170, 182,
337, 339
accidents, 24, 33, 48, 59, 85, 158,
173–77, 185, 211, 214, 216, 242,
244, 270, 275–77, 289
acetylcholine, 55
acidosis, 56–57, 77, 159, 194, 211,
227, 251, 279
Acute fatty liver of pregnancy, 318, 337
AD (Agitated delirium), 55–57
Adrenal Insufficiency, 177–78, 337
advanced age, 25, 143, 179, 183, 192,
201, 239
AFLP (Acute Fatty Liver of Pregnancy),
318
AIDS, 183, 258, 267, 279, 286
air bag fatalities, 184
alcohol, 54–56, 66, 68, 73, 75–85, 88,
91, 93, 135, 141, 175–78, 229,
233, 243, 245, 331–32
alcoholic cardiomyopathy, 82, 133, 135
alcoholic intoxication, acute, 26, 80,
141
Alcoholics Anonymous, 84
allergic reaction, acute. *See*
anaphylaxis
Ambien, 79

American Heart Association, 105,
111, 332
amiodarone, 97, 111, 165
amphetamines, 77–78, 84–85, 140,
191
amyloidosis, 146
anaphylaxis, 26, 185–87, 281,
338
anemia, hemolytic, 224
aneurysm, 25, 29–31, 34–38, 40–42,
71, 129, 162, 323, 338, 340, 344
abdominal aortic, 19, 30, 42, 179,
182, 203, 222, 247, 287, 337
coronary artery, 38, 131
sinus of valsalva, 41
splanchnic artery, 41–42, 348
angina pectoris, 202, 338, 340
angiogram, 33, 36, 38, 63, 97, 112,
125, 180, 323, 338
angiography, 37, 71, 91, 115, 127–28,
131, 264, 306, 338
anorexia, 26, 73, 155, 163, 191, 236
aorta, 29, 31–35, 37, 40, 42, 151, 158,
181, 198, 264, 306, 323, 339
abdominal, 34, 42, 337
aortic dissection, 19, 32–34, 91, 150,
222, 323, 339
aortic valve, 29, 34, 91, 121, 148–50,
152–53, 181, 246
appendicitis, 192, 265
ARVD (arrhythmogenic right
ventricular dysplasia), 147, 162,
190, 221, 300, 339

ABOUT THE AUTHOR

Eduardo Chapunoff, MD, is a diplomate of the American Board of Internal Medicine and the American Board of Cardiovascular Disease, a fellow of the American College of Physicians and the American College of Cardiology. He was a clinical associate professor of medicine at the University of Miami from 1985 to 1997.

He was the medical director of St. Francis Hospital Institute, Miami Beach, and the acting chief of staff at the Veterans Administration Outpatient Clinic, Oakland Park, Florida.

Dr. Chapunoff has been included in the biographical records of Marquis Who's Who Publication Board, Personalities of America, Community Leaders of America (American Biographical Institute), and the International Who's Who of Intellectuals (International Biographical Centre, Cambridge, England). He was named International Man of the Year 1991-1992 (International Biographical Centre, Cambridge, England).

He's the author of *Sex and the Cardiac Patient* **(1991)** and its Spanish version *El Sexo y el Paciente Cardiaco* **(1992),** which was also published in Argentina by Editorial Lidiun (1993). El Ateneo, one of the most prestigious publishing houses in South America, was its exclusive distributor. The English version was sold in countries as distant as Singapore and Australia.

In 2004 he published *Answering Your Questions about Heart Disease and Sex.* This work was designated as the **Editor's Choice** by iUniverse Publishing and was a *finalist* for *ForeWord Magazine's* **2004 Book of the Year Awards.** In October 2007, the book was published by **Hatherleigh, New York (distributor: Random House).**

In 2007, he published *Morbid Obesity and the Struggle for Survival* (**Editor's Choice** by iUniverse). This book has been revised and updated, and the new version is in print, with this title: *Morbid Obesity: Will You Allow it to Kill You?* (**Xlibris**)

How Not To Drop Dead! and the books on *Morbid Obesity and Heart Disease and Sex* are being translated into Spanish by the author himself and they are expected to become available to the public in the first half of 2010.

The Customer's Research Council of America-2009 named him one of "America's Top Cardiologists".

Dr. Chapunoff is currently the chief of cardiology at the Doctor's Medical Center and its six medical facilities, Miami, Florida.

His extracurricular activities include violin playing and oil painting. His artwork has been displayed in art galleries a number of times.

Visit his Web site: www.dreduardochapunoff.com

www.ingramcontent.com/pod-product-compliance
Lightning Source LLC
Chambersburg PA
CBHW031818170526
45157CB00001B/106